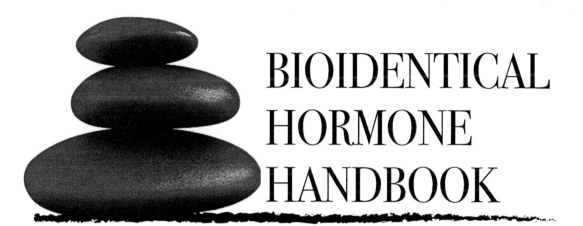

BIOIDENTICAL HORMONE HANDBOOK

Drs. Chris and Deanna Osborn

SECOND EDITION

A Word of Caution to the Reader

The information presented in this book is based on the training and professional experience of the authors. The treatments recommended in this book should not be undertaken without first consulting a physician. Proper laboratory and clinical monitoring is essential to achieving the goals of finding safe and natural treatments. This book was written for informational and educational purposes only. It is not intended to be used as medical advice.

Acknowledgements:

John Lee M.D. and David Zava Ph. D. for pioneering research and discoveries in the area of bio-identical hormone balancing and Eunice Van Winkle Ray for her tireless dedication to women's health and numerous editorial revisions and advice involved in completing this project.

Dedication:

Dr. Chris Osborn: For my beautiful wife , who introduced me to the concept of natural hormone balancing. Your efforts made this book possible. And your desire to help women achieve optimal health was the inspiration.

Dr. Deanna Osborn: We would like to dedicate this work to all women who are searching for answers to hormone balance and health for themselves as well as their families. It is our desire to bring awareness about environmental issues that affect our health to the forefront, so that we can make a lasting difference for generations to come.

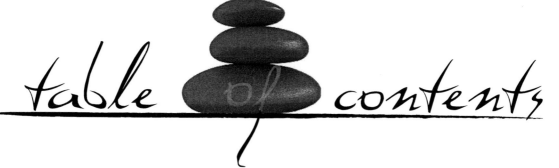

table of contents

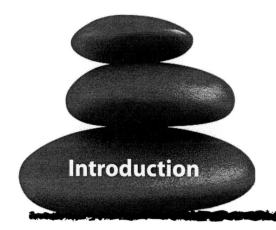

Introduction

It's not your fault…that's our message to you today. If you have ever lost control of your emotions, if for no apparent reason you have lashed out at the very people you love, if you have felt the pain and isolation of depression and chronic fatigue, or if your marriage has suffered from a libido that, well, isn't worth mentioning, then you are not alone. Do you feel like your monthly is more like your weekly? Do you wish your husband would have to feel your pain just once when you're suffering instead of him commenting, "Oh it's that time again huh?"

Well, be encouraged. We want to re-emphasize: It is not your fault. But there is a reason why you and many other women in the modern world feel this way. So whose fault is it then anyway? We should hang the person responsible!! How has this happened? And most importantly what in the world can we do about it? These are some of the questions we hope to answer for you in this handbook.

As family practice physicians, we have seen numerous women come into the office suffering from a multitude of complaints, and traditional treatments often times provided absolutely no relief. While traditional pharmaceutical-based modern medicine can be a life saver in some instances, there are instances when you have to look for answers beyond the scope of that context. In our journey to find answers to pressing health problems not adequately treated within the traditional medical model, we have learned a great deal and this book contains some of our findings which can be very helpful to many women today.

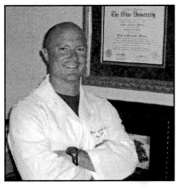

Dr. Chris Osborn

How has the modern woman found herself in such a horrible situation? A woman's body has been beautifully and wonderfully made. She boasts a balance of intricate and remarkable hormones, emotions, and physical capabilities with which her Maker most definitely must be pleased. If all things are as designed, she is capable of supplying love and strength to her spouse, birthing and nurturing her children, and providing bountifully from her wonderful store of gifts and talents to her friends, her family, and her community. Sadly, for too many, something has derailed her from the path set out by Nature for her optimal health, balance, and productivity. We intend to help you see, perhaps for the first time, how maybe, just maybe, you can begin to get back on track again.

We know first hand horomone imbalance issues as Deanna suffered from many of the symptoms listed above and more. It was not good for her or her family. When we married, Deanna was a picture of good health, but time and circumstances took their toll on her health. Even though we are both doctors, traditional medical approaches did not help her; in fact many made her feel worse. But her story ends well. Listen to her story.

Hi, I am Deanna Osborn and ten years ago, in 2002, at the age of 33, I was practicing medicine full time, but was very sick myself. I had struggled with joint pain since my teenage years. I remember waking up and wondering if I could even walk across the floor at the age of 17. I remember thinking "What will my life be like when I am old?!" I developed other symptoms like constipation, extremely dry skin and severe fatigue, chronic abdominal pain and lethargy which led to an eventual diagnosis of hypothyroidism at the age of 18.

Chris and I met and married while in medical school and our first child arrived during my fourth year of medical school; the second child came during my internship, and our third while doing my family practice residency. I am a "type A" personality who rarely knows her own limits. I point this out because it is this personality type that can literally wake up bewildered one day in a poor state of health and wonder, "How on earth did I get here?" I know because it happened to me.

I conveniently ignored the signs my body sent all along the way. After having my third child, I discovered my periods were so heavy I thought I was having a monthly miscarriage, though I knew this was not the case. I was also occasionally experiencing moderate to severe PMS. I didn't like who I was three days out of a month and neither did my family. It was as if I had a complete personality change.

Over the next two years not only did the bleeding get worse and worse, but I was diagnosed with psoriatic arthritis (an inflammatory type of arthritis similar to rheumatoid arthritis) by a local rheumatologist. I was told if I did not start taking a serious "disease modifying drug" I would be in a wheelchair in 10 years time.

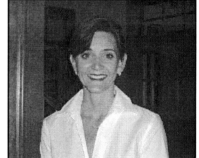

Delivering that diagnosis to me - a person who hit the floor running first thing in the morning and who continued in this mode all day until she fell into bed - was like issuing a death sentence. Reluctantly, I started the medication. A medication injected weekly with numerous side effects. While the arthritis pain improved, everything else seemed to deteriorate further.

Dr. Deanna Osborn

The most serious side effect of this medication was that it completely wiped out my immune system. I caught every cold, flu and strep throat that came my way and I had also developed some pretty severe gastrointestinal problems.

During this time, I was introduced to bioidentical progesterone by a close friend and patient, who knew of my heavy periods. The bleeding had become so severe that I was now very anemic. To manage my growing health issues, I had to often cancel patients because I just felt terrible. I tried everything conventional medicine and my profession had to offer and was ready to have a hysterectomy. As I looked at the bioidentical progesterone given to me by a non-medical friend, I decided I didn't have anything to lose so I tried the progesterone, applying it to my skin for transdermal absorption. To my amazement, it worked and worked very well. In fact, I could tell a difference at my very next cycle! After using it for three months, my periods became normal and to my further surprise and absolute delight, my PMS went away completely! From the time I started my period as a teen, I had always determined when my period would start based upon how I felt. It was the only time that I was ever grumpy.

I retested my blood work after three months of progesterone therapy to find that my anemia had been resolved and my thyroid function had improved. I kept asking myself, "Why didn't I know about this? Why isn't this being taught in medical schools? It's such a cheap and easy solution to so many women's issues." And that question began my personal education and relentless pursuit to find out everything I possibly could about bioidentical progesterone and its therapeutic uses. I was simply amazed at what I learned. This also opened my mind to a different approach to medicine than what I had been taught in medical school. It gave me permission, in a sense, to start thinking outside of the box, to start looking at health from a different perspective. To start looking for the root cause of the problem and not just take care of symptoms with a medication.

I was suffering from a pretty severe hormone imbalance called estrogen dominance/progesterone deficiency. It didn't happen overnight, but instead it was a gradual process, an incremental decline in my overall health. The ending to my story is very positive. I learned the absolute importance of proper diet, of using dietary supplements, and of the benefits of many herbs. I was able to see my hormones come into balance, my arthritis and GI issues resolve through the use of these supplements and herbs, and my overall health improved tremendously. Today I am in great health. As my health improved, Chris and I related my journey of recovery to the women in our medical practice. There were so many women coming to see us for PMS, depression, decreased sex drive, and so much more. Many patients unquestioningly rely upon birth control. However, many women of all ages - from teenagers to postmenopausal - may not fully understand the potential for negative outcomes associated with birth control use.

For example, there are many 30-40 somethings I have seen who experience classic symptoms related to their history of birth control pill use. The domino effect can look something like this: after taking birth control, migraine headaches can develop, then migraine medication is added to the birth control. Patients can became depressed from the effects of the birth control's high estrogen exposure, leading to a prescription for antidepressants. (I specifically remember being told by a psychiatrist, during one of my psychiatry rotations, that many mental illnesses would go away or be less complicated, if we could get people off of birth control pills. This was especially true among adolescents.) At this point, a patient may find they have absolutely no interest in sex. Often they gain weight, especially around the mid-section due to the estrogen they are ingesting via birth control. In addition, cravings for carbohydrates and refined sugars can become seemingly uncontrollable and lead to increased weight gain and high insulin levels. Due to the additional weight and chronically high levels of circulating insulin, patients can become insulin resistant and be at risk for diabetes and high blood pressure, both of which require treatment with more medications. At this point, in what is often a relatively short period of time, the patient often feels terrible; she's overweight, depressed, has migraines, no interest in sex, has been diagnosed with diabetes and hypertension, and is taking, on average, 5-9 medications! Sound familiar? It's then that she wakes up and says, "How did I get here?" Often it is a process so gradual that she hardly noticed. Is that the track that you are on? Or is that the track someone you know and care very much about is on?

We have access to so much more information than our parents and grandparents did. *The New England Journal of Medicine* states that "Preventable illness makes up approximately 70 percent of the burden of disease and the associated costs." There are so many great resources out there that can help you educate yourself and take control of your own health and wellness. Dig a little deeper and you can do this, just like we did! You won't learn everything overnight. It is a gradual process to return to health naturally. But, our promise to you is that you can begin to feel better in a week's time.

~Chris and Deanna

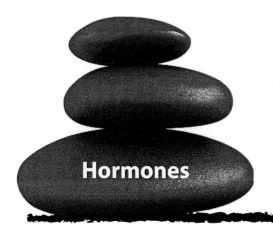

Hormones

Hormone imbalance is a condition that may affect a young lady early, even at the onset of menses. Years ago the average age when girls started their periods was about 16. Currently the average age at the onset of menstruation is right around 12. Exposure to environmental estrogens and the increasing amount of body fat in young adults is believed to play a role in this change. Body fat also produces estrogens and may increase the levels of these hormones circulating in the bloodstream.

Today over 50 percent of adolescent females experience some menstrual dysfunction. This may include dysfunctional uterine bleeding (abnormal menstruation either in the amount of bleeding or the frequency), amenorrhea (no menstruation), dysmenorrhea (painful menstruation), and premenstrual syndrome (PMS). Most are minor including mild cramping and pain with periods and minor variations in cycles. However, in some cases it can be severe and includes debilitating dysmenorrhea and severe abnormal uterine bleeding. In some cases, the bleeding may cause significant anemia from blood loss. About 45-70 percent of all post-pubescent females have some degree of dysmenorrhea, with up to 15 percent of these females describing the pain as severe and being incapacitated for 1-3 days per month.[1]

Hormonal imbalance affects 80 percent of U.S. women at peri-menopause (the time period before the cessation of the menstrual cycle, sometimes as early as thirty-five years of age) when disruptive and persistent symptoms can appear.[2] This can be very frustrating for a woman with this condition and also for her immediate family, her doctor and even her employer. Most women have an idea the symptoms they are experiencing seem to have a hormonal component because the symptoms often worsen with their menstrual cycle, but they don't know what to do about this condition, and quite honestly, most physicians do not know what to do with them either. Due to widespread misunderstanding, it is not uncommon for these women to be placed on birth control pills or antidepressant therapies, which in the long run can make the problem worse.

Some of the symptoms of hormonal imbalance are stress, acne, menstrual cramps, hair loss, PMS, fatigue, irritability, hot flashes, night sweats, migraine headaches, endometriosis, infertility, decreased sex drive, depression, weight gain, osteoporosis or osteopenia, dry skin, polycystic ovarian syndrome(PCOS), abnormal periods, heavy or painful periods, first trimester miscarriages, joint pain and breast cancer. Sounds like a lot of people you know, doesn't it? Hormone imbalance really is a condition that has reached epidemic proportions.

Unopposed Estrogen:

Continuous stimulation of the uterine lining with estrogen will lead to uterine cancer unless progesterone is also taken or used in conjunction with the estrogen. But, it is somewhat naïve to think that estrogen not balanced with progesterone will cause issues in only the uterus. Every cell in the body has both estrogen and progesterone receptors; therefore they BOTH play a role in every cell's function. For many years estrogens were prescribed to women for a variety of reasons without the addition of progesterone; and subsequently many women developed uterine cancer, which led to hysterectomy or even death. In this situation, we would say the uterine cancer is iatrogenic, or caused by a medical treatment. That's not to say that physicians caused the cancer intentionally, but they just didn't understand how vital the addition of progesterone was when prescribing estrogen. In medicine, progesterone was often considered just the pregnancy hormone, and not necessary for anything else. That is simply not the case! Now, at least, it is standard medical practice to prescribe progesterone with estrogens (albeit the synthetic versions). What continues to concern us is that many women, who have had their uterus and ovaries removed for whatever reason, are prescribed estrogen without progesterone, termed "unopposed estrogen". The flaw in this line of thinking is - what about all of the other tissues and organs that are exposed to alarmingly high levels of synthetic estrogen without the balancing protection of progesterone? Bottom line is I would not ever recommend taking estrogen alone! Your body was created to have both estrogen and progesterone present working together in harmony. If you are going to continue to take estrogens, your body needs to balance it with bioidentical progesterone.

Our bodies are very complex and the reproductive hormones are certainly a part of the mix! Women have many hormones that affect their reproductivity, but the focus of this handbook is primarily on estrogen and progesterone. No discussion of reproductive hormones would be complete however without mentioning the adrenal hormones and thyroid hormones, so included at the end of this handbook is a brief section on adrenal glands and thyroid hormones.

How Two Sex Hormones Work

Estrogen and progesterone are sex hormones made primarily in the ovaries. They work together so that a woman is able to have children, but when these two are out of balance, the effects can be devastating. Estrogen is the hormone that is most active during the first half of a woman's cycle. It is responsible for development of the egg and development of the lining of the uterus. At about the 14th day of a woman's cycle ovulation occurs. This is also when a woman will have an increase in progesterone levels. The mature egg has been released and the remnant of the egg, the corpus luteum, produces progesterone.

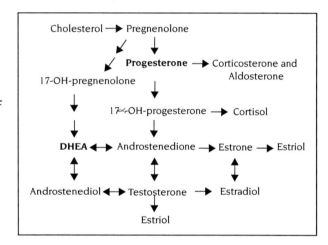

Progesterone is the pregnancy hormone. A woman cannot maintain a pregnancy without progesterone. If the corpus luteum is deficient, her body will not be able to maintain the endometrial lining or the fertilized egg. This deficiency is the most common cause of first trimester miscarriages and a symptom of a lack of progesterone. Progesterone is highly active in the 2nd half of the woman's cycle. It is responsible for maintaining the lining of the uterus so that the egg can implant. Progesterone has an opposing or "balancing" effect on estrogen, in effect sending the message that the endometrial lining can stop growing because it is sufficient for implantation of the egg.

It is during the 2nd trimester of pregnancy, after the 3rd month, that the placenta surrounding the baby is developed and takes over the function of progesterone production. During the last trimester of pregnancy the placenta will produce up to 400mg of progesterone a day. The average non-pregnant female only makes about 20mg per day.

In addition to its important reproductive aspects, progesterone is an important hormone in the fetal development of the central nervous system, including the brain. There are some recent studies that link progesterone to the development or repair of nerves. Our nerves are wrapped with a coating called myelin sheath. Myelin sheath is made up of cells called Schwann cells. It appears that progesterone stimulates the production of these Schwann cells. Given that our body was created with the amazing ability to repair or heal itself, it is reasonable to conclude that the stimulation/production of Schwann cells by progesterone is the bodies attempt to repair neurological damage.

It is very important for any woman considering the use of bioidentical hormones to maintain or achieve balance in her life to know or learn how her body works. Our bodies send so many "signals" which can be recognized, if we pay attention, but most of us either don't see the signals or don't understand what our bodies are saying to us. Since hormones fluctuate minute by minute in our system based upon stress, emotion, physical condition, etc., it is important that we learn to recognize those signals and respond appropriately. For example, there are times when a woman's body may only need to be supplemented with 20mg of USP Progesterone and there are stressful times when she will need 40mg of USP Progesterone per day. The woman who is tuned in and listening to her body can understand the signals more effectively and therefore better manage any hormonal imbalance. You need to know your body better than anyone else.

It is important to realize that, while we focus primarily on the use of bioidentical USP Progesterone in this handbook, there are often cases in which a woman is not only low in progesterone but also in estrogen. In that case, transdermal (applied to the skin) estrogen can be used. We have used transdermal estrogen in our practice in the form of Bi-est which is a combination of estradiol and estriol. These are two forms of estrogen often referred to in the literature as E1 and E3.

Estriol is the estrogen a woman makes during pregnancy and is the safest of the estrogens. Some studies show that it is actually estrogen metabolites that seem to stimulate cancer cells, not the estrogen. In a sense estriol is like a saturated fat. It cannot be oxidized into a metabolite which makes it a safer estrogen. Estrone is the strongest estrogen and potentially the most harmful. The subject of which estrogen to take is certainly an important one, but not one that we are covering in this handbook, but know this - estrogen should NEVER be taken by mouth, even if it is a bioidentical estrogen. The reason estrogen should not be taken by mouth is that as it passes through the liver it is metabolized into the more dangerous form of estrogen, estrone.

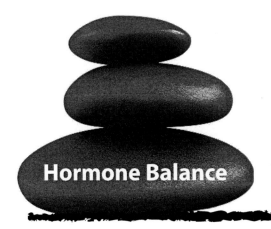

Hormone Balance

Hormones get out of balance through a variety of factors including dietary consumption of estrogens, lifestyle, medications, and even environment. Diet plays a big role. A diet high in carbohydrates or simple sugars actually makes hormonal imbalance worse. When you are consuming a diet high in carbohydrates your body's response is to have high circulating insulin levels. High insulin levels can be deletorious because insulin is a growth hormone and it is the only hormone in the body that causes us to store fat in our fat cells. Estrogen can actually be made in the fat by fat cells. A high carbohydrate diet will make you pack on weight around the waist in particular. All of this further contributes to hormone imbalance.

Life style is another big factor. Most of us are constantly on the go, trying feverishly to meet deadlines, pick up kids, run errands, and literally hold it all together! A person under a lot of stress will generally produce a lot of the cortisol hormone made by the adrenal glands. One of the building blocks of cortisol is progesterone. If you allow yourself to remain in a constant state of stress requiring high levels of cortisol, it will force your body to use up all of the progesterone to make cortisol. The body's hormones are interrelated and all must be balanced together.[3] High levels of cortisol are particularly deleterious to you, because over time it will interfere with your sleep cycles, shut down your immune system, and give you a significantly higher risk for developing cancers. This cycle is very taxing to the adrenal glands because that is where cortisol is made and will eventually lead to adrenal fatigue and/or failure.

Medications play a role in hormone imbalance. Some have the ability to wrongly bind to our body's natural hormone receptors, thereby blocking access for our beneficial hormones. Birth control pills and synthetic hormone replacement therapy (traditional hormone replacement therapy) play a huge role in blocking hormone receptors.

Sadly, many adolescents are prescribed birth control pills to control acne, treat PMS, to decrease amounts of bleeding during the menstrual cycle, to prevent pregnancy and even for the sake of convenience. Many are now given what is called "continuous birth control" which stops the menstrual cycle for a year. This is a very dangerous path to walk! Birth control pills completely control hormonal cycles with man-made hormones, completely shutting down a woman's natural hormone production. Use of birth control pills have been linked to breast cancer, and the longer a woman takes them the greater her risk. We are in an unprecedented time in medicine in which many women end

What is Fertility Awareness?

Searching for alternatives to birth control pills and patches has led to a great interest in Fertility Awareness. The Fertility Awareness Center of New York defines the Fertility Awareness Method (FAM) "as a body of knowledge by which a woman can know exactly when she is fertile and when she is not. With this knowledge, she can avoid pregnancy absolutely naturally, simply by not having unprotected intercourse when she is fertile. She can also use this information to help her achieve pregnancy and to gain insight into her health." FAM uses your basal body temperature (BBT), cervical fluid (CF), and changes in the cervix (CC) as the guideline for these determinations.

One of the most important factors in correctly using progesterone therapies is to know when to start the progesterone each month. To do this, determine when (or if) you ovulate via basal body temperature (BBT), cervical fluid (CF), and changes in the cervix (CC) to determine where you are in your menstrual cycle. FAM also teaches you how to read body signs as you approach ovulation. FAM is useful when incorporating progesterone therapies into your life, but is also an effective method of birth control and achieving pregnancy naturally. The skill doesn't replace the need to consult with medical professionals, but when used properly can assist you and your doctor in determining a course of action for a variety of health situations. After learning FAM you will understand how to chart your temperature, read your cervical fluid, and learn what your cervix is telling you. All of these different aspects will help you let your body lead you and your doctor in the direction that it wants or needs to go.

- Taking Charge of Your Fertility by Toni Weschler

up starting birth control at the age of 14, take it through their childbearing years, then transition to hormone replacement therapy for the menopausal years. Since the 1970s, many women have consumed artificial hormones for 30 years or more! Never has the use of synthetic hormones for this length of time been studied.

If you are the mother of a young daughter, we appeal to you to do some research of your own into the risks associated with birth control before walking this path with your adolescent. The risks are simply not worth it. These synthetic hormones are fakes. They are man-made attempts to mimic Mother Nature which simply cannot be done.

More troubling is that many people do not realize the hormones in pills, patches and vaginal rings are also being excreted in an active form in the urine of the women taking them. Those active forms make it to the waterways and eventually back to us. Along the way they cause significant damage to fish and other creatures living in our waterways. There are many studies that show 30 percent of male fish in lakes and rivers in the U.S. are able to produce eggs like a female. The scientists studying the fish contribute this trouble with reproductivity to the estrogens in the waterways. This issue is of great concern to us. Tighter regulations on these medications and better water treatment strategies are needed, or we can expect similar changes among our own species. It may not be as drastic as male animals producing eggs, but certainly decreased sperm counts in humans found by researchers today are being attributed to this cause. This is a much bigger and certainly a more pressing issue than global warming. The research is well documented and yet it seems to get little attention from our government and the media. Pharmaceutical and chemical companies have very deep pockets which can make it easy for watchdog agencies to look the other way.

We also cannot overlook the impact that our environment has on the issue of hormone imbalance. There are many chemicals in our environment that have the ability to bind to estrogen receptors and create an unwanted effect in the body. Pesticides, plastics, household cleaning products, cosmetic products that are petroleum-based or that contain mineral oil, herbicides, fungicides and the list goes on. These compounds that are able to bind to receptors and interfere with our natural hormones are often referred to as xenoestrogens or "false estrogen." To say that we are swimming in a sea of estrogen would be a very accurate description!

Understanding the Difference Between
Bioidentical Hormones and Synthetic Hormones

The difference between the way synthetic hormones and bioidentical hormones work in the body is like the difference between night and day! A synthetic hormone is a man-made version, or copycat of what the body makes, but not exactly. While the synthetic version may have some of the same effects as the "real deal" it comes with many adverse side effects.

The biochemical composition of a bioidentical hormone is identical to what our human bodies make, so when we use the phrase bioidentical USP Progesterone, we are referring to progesterone that is exactly like what the body makes on its own. A great deal of the confusion in this matter exists because of the confusion in the medical field. The difference is simply not taught in medical schools. Progesterone is viewed as the same thing as progestin (the term for the synthetic version). It is wrong to view them from this perspective because the chemical composition is so different! Progesterone actually supports and maintains pregnancy. However, synthetic progestins are absolutely contraindicated during pregnancy and may cause serious birth defects. Quite a difference!

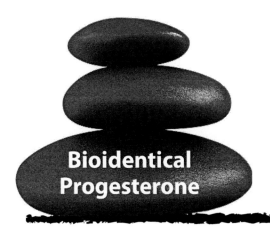

Bioidentical Progesterone

Progesterone Supplements

To use progesterone properly, it is important to understand how a woman's cycle works. The average woman will have a 28-day menstrual cycle, but most women are not average and will find that their actual cycle is a little shorter or a little longer. In a 28-day cycle, day 1 of the cycle is the day you start to bleed. Day 14 is when you ovulate and then day 28 is the day before you start your period. The only thing that is consistent in a woman's cycle is that 14 days after she ovulates, if she is not pregnant, she will start to menstruate.

When a woman ovulates is often the tricky part. For some it is on day 8; for others it might be day 16! When ovulation occurs we see a peak in progesterone levels. It appears that this peak is in part what is responsible for the woman's increased sex drive during ovulation. Some women will feel a slight cramping in their low abdomen associated with ovulation. Most women will experience a slight discharge that

Note from Deanna -
Eighty percent of women can achieve hormone balance using progesterone therapy. I cannot say that it will work for everyone because many people have more complex issues. Often the thyroid is involved or the adrenals are overstressed. Many times they are on so many medications that it is difficult to tell if they are experiencing a symptom from a disease or a side effect from a medication. The following section will cover how I have used progesterone in my medical practice for the treatment of various female problems.

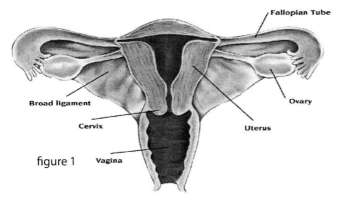

figure 1

Labels on figure: Fallopian Tube, Broad ligament, Cervix, Ovary, Uterus, Vagina

is clear, stringy and odorless. The clear, stringy nature of the discharge is often described as having an egg white-like consistency. After the woman ovulates the egg makes its way to the fallopian tube (see figure 1) where it may or may not be fertilized. If it is fertilized, the egg will implant into the woman's uterine lining where it will start to grow and develop. If the egg is not fertilized, the endometrial lining of the uterus will start to slough off, which is the start of the woman's period. Over and over and over this process happens 12 times a year, or, on average, 444 times during her reproductive life! All women need to read and learn about how their bodies work. Investigating fertility awareness is one way to begin your learning curve.

Evaluating a Progesterone Product

There are a few things that are important to look for in finding a progesterone product. It is important to find progesterone that is bioidentical and USP Progesterone, which means it meets United States Pharmacopeia standards. Bioidentical simply means that one molecule of progesterone from the product would look exactly like a molecule of progesterone in a woman's body. USP guarantees that you are actually getting progesterone in the bottle and not just a soy cream or a wild yam cream. The product should be in an airtight container so that it is not being continually oxidized by air. Avoid using progesterone that comes in a jar from which you scoop out the product by hand. You should also look at the base ingredients with which the progesterone was mixed to make sure that there is no mineral oil. Mineral oil can interfere with the body's ability to appropriately absorb progesterone. It's also a petrochemical and we do not recommend using skin care products that contain it. USP Progesterone is readily available within the marketplace and can easily be obtained through a local health food store, compounding pharmacy, or health and wellness company.

Bone Health

It is important to realize that progesterone is only part of the picture in bone health. You also have to look at Vitamin D levels. It is well known and accepted that we need to take extra calcium but not many people realize that we are actually deficient in Vitamin D. When you look at the recommended daily amount of Vitamin D in our society, you need to know that it was established based on the amount of Vitamin D required to prevent rickets. Most of us are deficient and should correct this.

I recommend testing of Vitamin D levels to help guide therapy. Generally taking 4000 to 8000 IU per day is acceptable. Twenty minutes of sun exposure per day without sunscreen, will allow your body to make about 10,000 IU of Vitamin D.

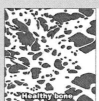 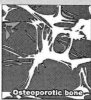

Healthy bone | Osteoporotic bone

Hormone Testing

It is important to understand that in many cases hormones being tested in the venous blood do not give a true picture of what is going on in the body. A vast majority (up to 99 percent) of the sex hormones are carried in the blood via sex hormone binding globulin (SHBG). This is the inactive (storage) form of the sex hormones. The free hormone which is not bound to the SHBG is the active form. It is bound to fatty substances because it is totally insoluble in water. This active form is not measured in the serum because the fatty substances are "spun off" in the centrifuge in processing the blood for testing. The best way to test hormones is either through a saliva hormone test or through a "blood spot" test (3). The free active form of sex hormones is easily tested in a saliva test or a peripheral tissue "blood spot" test via a finger prick. Saliva and blood spot testing are dependable and becoming more widely used. You can have a saliva test or blood spot test done through ZRT labs in Beaverton, Oregon (www.ZRTlabs.com). Saliva testing is great for checking hormone levels as well as cortisol levels. The blood spot, a simple finger prick, can be used to check hormone levels, thyroid levels, insulin levels, Vitamin D levels and much more.

How do I use progesterone cream? To use transdermal bioidentical USP Progesterone cream, apply via the skin. Massage into hands, feet, inner arms, neck, chest, breasts and/or abdomen. Rotate the sites with each use.

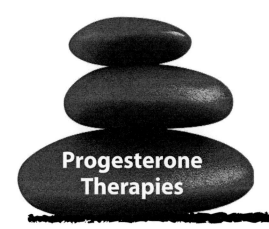

Progesterone Therapies

Using Progesterone for Endometriosis

Endometriosis is a painful female condition that can have a negative impact on one's ability to become pregnant. It can cause heavy and painful periods as well. The exact cause of endometriosis is unknown but what happens in this disease is that pieces of the endometrial lining (lining of the uterus) are outside of the uterus. The pieces are often called "endometrial implants" and they may attach themselves to the inside of the abdomen, the ovaries, the colon and even the fallopian tubes. Most women experience severe cramping with their period when they have endometriosis.

We recommend patients use 20-30mg of USP Progesterone daily for endometriosis. It is best to break the dose in half and use 10mg in the morning and 10-20mg in the evening. We also recommend using it all month long except when menstruating. It is best to follow these guidelines for about 3-4 months. At that time, if the woman is doing better and noticing a decrease in symptoms, we recommend that she start using progesterone on days 12-26 of her cycle (this is assuming she has a normal 28-day cycle).

Using Progesterone for PCOS (Polycystic Ovarian Syndrome) or PCOD (Polycystic Ovarian Disease)

PCOS is a condition that affects the ovaries with the development of multiple cysts on the ovaries. The ovaries become diseased and infertility may become an issue. There is a metabolic component to PCOS as well. High levels of carbohydrates and simple sugars stimulate the body to produce high levels of insulin. Insulin will stimulate the production of androgens (male hormones). Many of these women will also suffer from facial hair and acne due to the excessive male hormones often produced. It is common place to treat PCOS with oral diabetic medications to reduce the levels of insulin. It would be much wiser and safer to treat the problem through strict diet, eliminating simple carbs and refined sugars, and supplementing with progesterone. We recommend patients use 20-30mg USP progesterone daily for 90 days. Stop after 90 days and menstruation should occur. Start using 20mg daily on days 12-26 of the menstrual cycle. At this point women should be having regular periods. Many women with PCOS who are trying to get pregnant can conceive as early as month 4.

Using Progesterone for PMS

PMS can be a debilitating condition for so many women and those around them. It is surprising how common the problem is and we believe it has so much to do with the excess estrogen in the environment to which women are exposed. Too often antidepressants are the therapeutic response used by traditional medicine. Sometimes antidepressants are prescribed for the entire month and sometimes only prescribed for the week of PMS. The problem with antidepressants is the lengthy side effect profile that can lead to the use of additional medications. We recommend patients use 20-30mg of USP Progesterone for the treatment of PMS. Progesterone will mainly address the mood swings, irritability and anxiety associated with PMS. Most women find progesterone works well for them when they use it on days 12-26 of their cycle, just before ovulation. For example, women who ovulate earlier than day 14 of their cycle, may want to start using it 2 days prior to ovulation. For a woman who normally ovulates on day 10, she should start using progesterone on day 8. This form of progesterone dosing is referred to as cyclical because it is designed to mimic what your body does naturally.

Using Progesterone for Abnormal Bleeding

Abnormal bleeding requires some special considerations. Any woman experiencing abnormal uterine bleeding (sometimes called dysfunctional uterine bleeding) should see a doctor first before trying progesterone. Although this is a very common problem due to hormonal imbalance, abnormal bleeding can also be a sign of endometrial cancer. Once endometrial cancer has been ruled out, then 20-30mg USP Progesterone can be used on days 12-26 of the menstrual cycle.

Using Progesterone for Infertility

Bioidentical progesterone can be used for female infertility, when the issue is anovulation or she is not ovulating. Progesterone is a widely accepted treatment for anovulation among fertility specialists. Generally, if a woman is not ovulating, it is because she has low progesterone levels. She may or may not have a period.

It is best to start out by using 20-40mg of USP Progesterone daily for 90 days, if you are not having a period. After the 90 days, stop using the progesterone and wait for a period. Once your period starts, begin using the progesterone on day 12 (of an average 28-day cycle) through the start of your menstrual cycle. While most women do not have a 28-day cycle, we will use the 28-day cycle as a model in this book. The following guidelines are based on the average 28-day cycle and may need adjusting for your particular cycle length.

For women not ovulating, but who are having a period, use 20-30mg of USP Progesterone on day 12 through the start of your period. The reason we recommend using the progesterone through the start of your period is that, if you are pregnant, the last thing we want to do is decrease the progesterone level. Some women with low progesterone levels suffer from frequent first trimester miscarriages. When an egg is fertilized just after ovulation it is the remnant that the egg leaves behind in the ovary, called the corpus luteum that produces progesterone. It produces progesterone for the entire first trimester. During the second and third trimester the placenta takes over and produces large quantities of progesterone. If a woman is low in progesterone, there is a high likelihood that she will miscarry during the first trimester. This is why it is important to keep the progesterone level constant through the start of your period. Once you start your period you can stop using the progesterone and begin again at day 12 of the cycle. If you do not start your period, take a pregnancy test. If it is positive, continue using the progesterone. If you have had a first trimester miscarriage in the past, it is best to increase the progesterone which is further discussed in the next section.

Using Progesterone for First Trimester Miscarriage

If you have suffered from a first trimester miscarriage or know a woman who has, you know how devastating it can be. Many women are plagued with multiple first trimester miscarriages due to a low progesterone level. Please read the previous section on progesterone use for infertility. If you have had a first trimester miscarriage in the past and want to use progesterone in an attempt to prevent it from happening again, We recommend to patients using 40-60mg of transdermal USP Progesterone daily the moment you find out you are pregnant. If you are already using progesterone when you get pregnant it is best to increase it to the 60mg daily, if you have a history of first trimester miscarriages. It is not necessary to use the transdermal progesterone for the entire pregnancy. At about the 16th week of pregnancy the placenta starts to produce large quantities of progesterone. It is acceptable at this point to stop using the transdermal progesterone. By the last trimester the placenta produces up to 400mg of progesterone a day! Remember this hormone is not only critical to maintain a pregnancy, but it also is very important in the development of the baby's central nervous system.

Using Progesterone for Osteopenia or Osteoporosis

Many women have bone loss over time without even realizing it and can greatly suffer with the results. The healthcare statistics on dollars spent treating osteoporosis and the subsequent effects are staggering. The good news is progesterone actually stimulates osteoblasts, cells within the bone that build bone. Many women using progesterone therapy will see improvements in their bone density tests over time. For maintaining bone health, we recommend 10mg USP Progesterone topically per day.

Using Progesterone for Postpartum Depression

Postpartum depression can be a very serious condition with life-threatening consequences for both the new mother and baby. Women with PMS have a higher risk of developing postpartum depression. Progesterone is safe for use in the postpartum period and while breast feeding. What we have witnessed to be effective in the treatment of postpartum depression is 20mg of transdermal USP Progesterone daily applied at night. Since progesterone has a calming effect it can help with insomnia and anxiety as well.

Using Progesterone for Depression, Anxiety and Insomnia

Many women in the U.S. have been improperly placed on antidepressant therapies when actually the root cause of their problem is hormone imbalance. When depression gets worse during the menstrual cycle or just before the cycle begins, it is a strong indication that a hormonal component exists. We recommend using 20mg USP Progesterone transdermally daily. It is best used at night because it can help with any sleep issues. An additional 10 to 20mg of progesterone can be used anytime during the day to treat anxiety.

Progesterone can also be used in conjunction with antidepressant therapy. Many women come to us and want to get off of their antidepressant medication. This always needs to be done with the assistance of their physician. We usually have them start using the progesterone and reevaluate their depressive symptoms 2-3 months later. At that point, if they are doing well, we would consider tapering off their antidepressant medication.

Using Progesterone for Decreased Libido or Low Sex Drive

Often women on progesterone therapy will notice an increase in sex drive. This is often because their hormones come back into balance with the progesterone and their body is actually able to use progesterone to make a small amount of testosterone through one of the many biochemical hormonal pathways. Testosterone works to increase sex drive and progesterone can also help to balance the adrenals, if the person is experiencing adrenal fatigue. Reducing mental and physical stress on the body is critical to overall health and reducing stress and the resulting adrenal fatigue can itself cause an increase in sex drive.

Using progesterone for menopausal symptoms

Many women who were on synthetic HRT (Hormone Replacement Therapy) wanted to discontinue it after the important Women's Health Initiative study results were released in 2002. The Women's Health Initiative study proved that using synthetic estrogens and progestins lead to an increase in stroke, heart attack and breast cancer. It is, in fact, recommended by the FDA that if a woman needs to use HRT that it should be for the shortest time period possible. We also know that the combination of nonbioidentical estrogen and progestin absolutely increases ones risk of developing dementia and lung cancer.

We have seen good results helping women cope with menopausal symptoms and titrating off of HRT with the use of bioidentical USP Progesterone. Progesterone can help with many menopausal symptoms. Specifically it can relieve hot flashes, vaginal dryness, mood swings, and irritability. It is the sudden decrease in estrogen that causes a woman to experience hot flashes or night sweats. Progesterone can be used by the body to make a small amount of estrogen, if the body needs it. Helene Leonetti, M.D., in a double-blind study of progesterone cream that was published in the journal Obstetrics and Gynecology in 1999, showed that menopausal symptoms such as hot flashes responded very nicely to progesterone cream in 83 percent of the women, while only 19 percent of women using the placebo got relief.[4]

Progesterone as an Alternative to HRT

If a woman is currently on an HRT and wants to get off of it, we recommend that she start using 20-30 mg of progesterone daily for a month in addition to her HRT. In the second month cut the pill in half while continuing with the transdermal progesterone. In month 3, decrease the HRT pill to 1/2 a pill every other day while using the progesterone and then discontinue the HRT in month 4. During this entire time, we have her use 20mg-30mg of USP Progesterone transdermally, all month with a 5 day break each month. There are some progesterone products that will include some phytoestrogens or plant estrogens that can also be very beneficial in resolving hot flashes. It is of benefit to take the 5 day break each month in an attempt to let the progesterone receptor sites down regulate or clear out. This will allow the product to work at a higher efficacy. Another option is to switch from the pill to a patch form of estrogen for the tapering-off period. Many women, after hearing about the WHI, stopped taking their Premarin or Prempro cold turkey. Many were miserable in doing this and suffered severe hot flashes and other symptoms. This is not necessary and can be avoided if the woman tapers off of her HRT and supplements with bioidentical progesterone. If a woman gets good results with this approach we usually recommend that she continue using the progesterone. If she is using a product with plant estrogens and is doing fine in terms of symptoms a year later, she can switch to using just USP Progesterone.

Using Progesterone for Uterine Fibroid Tumors

Estrogen is the "food supply" that causes fibroid tumors to grow. What women need to know is that fibroid tumors NEVER turn into cancer, but shrink and go away with the onset of menopause. The reason is simple. The "food supply" or estrogen levels decline once you start menopause. The problem with fibroid tumors is that they can contribute to heavy bleeding and painful periods. Although it has not been proven, we believe that since progesterone opposes the action of estrogen it is conceivable that regular progesterone use over time would in fact decrease the size of a fibroid tumor. This is an area of progesterone therapy we have wanted to study for quite some time, after clinically seeing women with fibroids substantially improve. We recommend using 20mg of progesterone daily or cyclically (day 14 – 28) for fibroid tumors.

Using Progesterone for Fibrocystic Breast Disease

Fibrocystic breast disease is a symptom of too much estrogen in the system and it seems to affect mainly women of child bearing years. Progesterone is an easy answer for treatment, because it opposes the action or blocks the action of estrogen at the cell. These women suffer from very tender or painful breast tissue that may or may not worsen at certain times in their menstrual cycle. The breast tissue is not only tender it also may feel lumpy to the touch. Many of these women feel what they think is a "mass" and end up with needle biopsy to find out that the mass is a cyst. The response to progesterone is pretty rapid and many women can tell a difference in 1-3 months. Using 20mg of progesterone daily or cyclically will usually alleviate the problem.

Menstrual Migraines

Some women experience migraine headaches that are cyclical in nature. Cyclical migraines are definitely hormone-related. They are usually due to excess estrogen and can be alleviated with the regular use of progesterone and usually 10-20mg of transdermal progesterone daily is usually sufficient to alleviate them. The progesterone can be used all month except for when menstruating or it can be used is a cyclical fashion to more closely mimic what a normal cycle would do. To use it cyclically, use 10-20 mg on days 12-26 of your cycle.

Using Progesterone in Breast Cancer

There is much controversy on this topic, but after much research and inquiry we agree that progesterone is breast protective. If you or a loved one has been diagnosed with breast cancer or is a breast cancer survivor, we strongly recommend that you read Dr. John Lee's and David Zava, PhD's book, *What Your Doctor May Not Tell You About Breast Cancer.* They point out much of the controversy in this area stems from the medical community's confusion between progestin and progesterone. Again, progestin is a synthetic, man-made version of progesterone. They are not the same hormone at all. Progestins are classified by the International Agency for Research on Cancer (IARC) as possibly carcinogenic to humans.[5] Progesterone is the hormone that all women make in their own bodies and for which there are receptors on every cell in our body whether it be a brain cell, a bone cell, a breast cell, etc!

Note from Deanna -
If there was one piece of information that I could pass along to every woman, man and every clinician it is this; be knowledgeable of a study on the timing of breast surgery during menstrual cycle. It has been shown that women who have their surgery during the luteal phase (progesterone phase) have a 2X greater overall survival rate. Remember from our previous discussion the luteal phase is the 2nd half of a woman's menstrual cycle.[6]

If you were a woman with breast cancer wouldn't you want to know that you can double your rate of survival just by selecting the timing of surgery?! Please take the time to look at the resources that I have included to support this position at the back of the book.

It is so important that we as a society and medical community stop confusing these two. Bioidentical progesterone and non bioidentical progestin cannot be lumped together. When looking at the biochemical structure of progesterone, it more closely resembles testosterone than it does progestin! Yet we know how different progesterone is from testosterone! It has become clear to us that when a woman is diagnosed with an estrogen positive and progesterone positive breast cancer that the progesterone receptors are the body's natural attempt to ward off or get rid of that cancer! It has been shown that a woman with a progesterone deficiency has a 10 fold increase risk of all malignant neoplasms compared to a woman without a progesterone deficiency.

It is also critical that any woman concerned with reducing breast cancer risk understand the importance of adrenal gland function. If a woman has high cortisol levels at night (which may be seen with adrenal fatigue) she will not be able to make melatonin. She will likely also suffer from insomnia or is just not able to go to bed until well after midnight. She probably feels like she can't even get out of bed in the morning. The problem with this is that melatonin stimulates the production/activation of Natural Killer Cells (NKC). NKC are cancer scavengers within our body. A woman with compromised adrenal glands, who has a suppressed cortisol level all day long and a higher cortisol level at night is putting herself at risk for cancer. We are including a section on adrenal fatigue and thyroid disease because it is critical to overall health.

Adrenal Fatigue

Adrenal fatigue is a condition that can often interfere with hormone balance. We as physicians have greatly underestimated the role of the adrenal glands. In medical school we are primarily taught that it either works or it doesn't; end of story. This is simply not the case and, as with many disease processes, there is a progression of the disease. To categorize it as working or non working, is too simplistic. Similar to diabetes, there is a continuum of the disease and variations of the disease. Some of the symptoms of adrenal fatigue are feeling tired in the morning, fatigue not relieved by sleep, increased effort to do daily tasks, craving salty foods, lethargy, decreased ability to handle stress and decreased sex drive. Additional symptoms can include depression, increased time to recover from illness, injury or trauma, feeling light-headed when you stand up quickly, less enjoyment or happiness with life, symptoms worsen when you skip meals, decreased tolerance, memory less accurate, fuzzy thinking and more! James

Wilson's book, *Adrenal Fatigue – The 21st Century Stress Syndrome* completely explains adrenal fatigue and treatment. If you have any of the above mentioned symptoms, please get a copy of that book and educate yourself. Sometimes many symptoms of adrenal fatigue and female hormonal imbalance can overlap. So it is essential to determine whether or not you may be suffering from this condition to achieve optimal balance.

Thyroid Disorders

It seems that the standard approach to diagnosing and treating thyroid disorders is a bit erroneous in traditional medicine too. Traditionally we are taught to measure a TSH (thyroid stimulating hormone) and if it is within normal range the person is normal. It seems a majority of patients will read the symptoms of low thyroid, come to the office to get checked for the disease only to be told they are "normal." They don't typically feel normal though. The problem with this test is it does not check what is going on in the thyroid or in the tissues! TSH tells us that the brain is functioning, but what about the thyroid gland? Too many times people can even present with a goiter of their thyroid gland and are told they are "normal" because their TSH is fine.

One problem with this type of thinking is explained in the way lab test "normals" are created. Scientists create a range of what is normal for a population by testing a large group of people from all age ranges. Ninety-five percent of the population will have an average TSH between 0.4 and 4.5, for example. In general, the lower the TSH the higher the thyroid levels in the bloodstream. However, as we age our thyroid function often declines and people who have a deficient thyroid are also included in the measurement. So, as a result, the so-called "normal" can be off. We should always strive for a TSH around 1.0, which is closer to the value seen in people with a youthful, fully functional thyroid gland. It is also critical to check a free T4 level, free T3 level, thyroid antibodies and sometimes a thyroid binding globulin. These thyroid function markers can be checked with traditional blood work or through the blood spot method mentioned earlier. If the thyroid antibodies are elevated, even if your thyroid markers are otherwise normal, you may have early autoimmune thyroid disease. T4 is the precursor form of thyroid hormone. That is what is found in the prescription medication Synthroid®. It has four iodine molecules on it, thus T4. The body converts T4 to T3 by cleaving off one of the iodine molecules. Before thyroid hormone can be utilized by the peripheral tissues and perform its functions, it must be converted to T3. Some people have trouble converting free T4 to T3 and this can be the problem that is causing their symptoms. If a woman seeks to balance her hormones, she must make sure that her thyroid hormones are in balance and adrenal glands are functioning properly. Otherwise hormone balance can forever elude her.

Problem Skin and Hormones

Skin "problems" are often the physical evidence of toxins moving through the body to be eliminated via the skin, the body's largest detoxifying organ. We often look for a little dab of medicinal fix-it to paint on a blemish to quickly remedy an unsightly pimple, but pimples erupting on the skin may signal something larger going on in body systems which may require more than topical skin treatments.

Skin problems let us know that hormones are out of balance, or that foods may be unmanageable by our body, and/or toxins are brimming to the top and spilling over onto the skin because the liver, the largest internal detoxifying system, is overloaded. Problem skin alerts us to malfunctions in the body, thereby signaling us to take remedial steps to avoid larger problems with body systems.

Forty to 50 million people in U.S. have acne. While acne is considered to plague only teenagers, many people over the age of 25 suffer from acne; 54 percent of women and 40 percent of men have some degree of acne, and children as young as 4 years old have been diagnosed. U.S. consumers spend $100 million in over-the-counter acne remedies per year to treat their symptoms. But what causes acne? Is it possible to "cure" acne if we treat the cause? The answer is yes.

According to Dr. Loren Cordain, acne is a result of the combination of diet and hormones which effect the skin's life cycle. Certain popular foods can increase androgens (male hormones) in the blood, causing the body to produce more oil, or sebum. Overproduction of sebum in pores contributes to acne, causing bacteria to colonize, which raises the level of inflammation and infection. The immune system kicks in and produces pro-inflammatory hormones called cytokines, resulting in a papule, pustules, or nodule (bumps, spots, or zits). In essence, the body's entire delicate balance of hormores is thrown out of sync by a chain reaction linked to diet.

The food culprits that trigger this domino effect are not limited to a single food group. Diets heavy in carbohydrates contribute to the delay in cell death (apoptosis), because carbohydrates rapidly increase insulin levels in the body. Carbohydrates can also be high glycemic-load foods, which elevate androgens in the blood stream and, as we have noted, created an overabundance of oil produced by the skin. Moreover, the Harvard School of Public Health demonstrated that milk so common to the American diet was associated with acne in a group of 47,355 women in the Nurse's Health Study. Hormones can be disrupted as the body breaks down the foods we don't necessarily need, like milk, but it is also possible to consume hormones directly from the milk that we drink. Milk also has the abilty to impair zinc absorption, a necessary nutrient in the skin's arsenal of defenses. Dairy products also induce high levels of insulin, leading to the same

Dr. Cordain, in his book The Dietary Cure for Acne contends with dermatology by declaring diet to be a causal factor for acne. Citing recent research, Dr. Cordain gives direction for what food groups to eliminate, because people with skin issues often have food sensitivities, are toxic and/or have hormones out of balance. Cordain also recommends eliminating foods that contribute to candida growth largely due to antibiotic overuse which can contribute to skin breakouts.

Detoxing and balancing hormones are the two first steps to regaining overall health and healthy skin, but eating clean is also necessary to optimum results in any health and skin regimen.

Action Items:
Diet: Dr. Cordain recommends eating lean meats and other proteins and low-sugar vegetables and eliminating dairy, nuts, sugar and carbs from your diet for a month. After a month, then add one food group back in to your diet to see if there are reactions to those foods on the skin.

Hormones: Your hormone baseline can be determined with a saliva test from ZRT Labs. Test kits are available online and are sent back to ZRT for reading. Balancing hormones with a bioidential hormone cream is an excellent first course and may be all that is needed. 20 mg of bioidential progesterone daily assists in hormone balancing. Use a light tight, air-tight pump container that dispenses 20mg with each pump.

Detoxing: Use of a 7 day body cleanse system each month for 3-4 months would be desirable and massage with antioxidant and mineral rich lotions and botanical oils to restore needed minerals; and to move the lymph system where wastes from the cells – carbon dioxide, lactic acid and metabolites – are carried back to the bloodstream through the lymph fluid.

sequence of events caused by carbohydrates, ultimately leading to acne.
In addition to carbohydrates, fats can cause a number of responses related to acne. Americans consume ten times more omega-6 than omega-3 oils (10:1), while the ideal ratio of omega-6 to omega-3 is 2:1. This 10:1 ratio produces a constant pro-inflammation in many body tissues, resulting in an immune response to invading bacteria perpetuating the acne cycle.

Prostate Problems

Like women, men make all three sex hormones: estrogen, progesterone and testosterone. Prostate cancer occurs in part because testosterone and progesterone levels fall with age and estrogen levels rise, leading to estrogen dominance in older men. Similar mechanisms that cause breast cancer and uterine cancer in women cause prostate cancer in men. Prostate problems are the fastest-growing health concern in Westernized countries; and the rate of prostate cancer is increasing steadily. Causal factors are thought to include estrogen dominance, testosterone deficiency, lack of sexual activity, zinc deficiency and insufficient nighttime sleep. A good night's sleep is so vital to health for so many reasons, but as mentioned previously is the effect of melatonin on natural killer cells (NKC). NKC are immune cells that seek out and kill any precancerous cells in the body. NKC activity is stimulated by the hormone melatonin[7] which is produced primarily while you are in a deep sleep. So not only should we get our beauty rest for good looks, but also for good health.

Dr. Eugene Shippen says testosterone is one key substance in the body that is more powerful than any other health factor and is more closely linked to risk of illness if and when deficiency occurs. Testosterone is more misunderstood, more improperly used, and more tragically underused than any other hormone. I have studied testosterone, prescribed it and watched the responses of my patients - hundreds of them. I challenge anyone to find a more diversely positive factor in men's health. When normally abundant, it is at the core of energy, stamina, and sexuality. When deficient, it is the core of disease and early demise.

The Testosterone Syndrome: The Critical Factor for Health, Energy and Sexuality - Reversing the Male Menopause

Estradiol in particular is harmful to a man's prostate because it causes the prostate to enlarge and likely is one of the main causes of prostate cancer. Progesterone inhibits the conversion of testosterone to di-hydro-testosterone (DHT) just like the drug, Proscar® and Saw Palmetto. Only progesterone is a much more potent inhibitor of this detrimental conversion. Higher levels of DHT and lower levels of testosterone are associated with prostate enlargement (BPH), prostate cancer and balding. Therefore, progesterone could benefit in all these conditions. Five to 10 mg of bioidentical progesterone each day is helpful in balancing the increasing estrogens in a man's body and will also assist in maintaining bone strength.

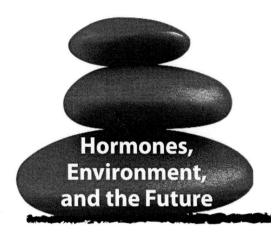

Hormones, Environment, and the Future

We hear a good deal about "the environment" today, but most of us don't realize how close pollution is to us nor do we understand the current and future implications for a petrochemical-based society which represents most of the developed world. We began following the news reports and conducting ressearch on the largely unseen hormone aspects of "pollution."

Toxin Exposure

There are thousands of studies that show the adverse hormonal effects of petrochemical pollutants which originate outside the body, but which find their way inside the body through drinking water, the air we breathe, and the lotions, creams and make-up we put on our skin. These pollutants disrupt the delicate endrocine system which manages the glands that make brain hormones, reproductive hormones, adrenal hormones, as well as insulin and thyroid hormones. For simplified discussion here, these endrocine disrupters can also have an estrogen-like effect upon the body. Some or all of a woman's hormone imbalance may be due to these factors. The concern over these environmental pollutants is the effect they have upon the reproductive organs of all living creatures. False estrogens are fat-soluble and nonbiodegradable and easily pass through the skin to be stored in body fat. There are some solutions to the problem so start with paying attention to the foods you eat. Animals are fattened up with hormones and eat grains grown with pesticides. These hormones and pesticides are stored in the animal's fat, and that your best to buy organic grass-fed meat, organic vegetables and drink filtered water.

Male Fish Making Eggs

In 2003 we noticed a news story about a little environmental fish study. The report then was that 30 percent of male fish in the Potomac River were able to produce eggs, quite obviously a female fish function.

In 2010, the follow up appeared on that same study. The research then showed that nearly 80 percent of the male fish in the Potomac River were able to produce eggs! The researchers concluded in 2003 and again in 2010, that the male fish are being feminized due to exposure to chemicals that include synthetic hormones (birth control and hormone replacement therapy – excreted into the water system and then into lakes and streams) as well as the run off into waterways from feed lots where livestock excrete growth hormones; and also the use of industrial and chemicals components found in plastics, fertilizers, insecticides, fungicides etc., which are also making their way into the streams and rivers from which the public water supply is drawn.

The Potomac Conservancy as well as the US Geological Survey followed this and other similar studies. In 2010, the US geological survey found "intersex" fish in a third of 111 sites tested around the country as powerful chemicals make their way into our waterways and greatly alter the natural function of life; and, uniformly, the finger of blame seems to unfailingly point to birth control pills as the primary culprit

Submerged in EDCs

In short, this is the environmental dilemma we are in today: Too much estrogen and other growth hormones which make it very difficult to balance one's hormones, but there is more to the story. As scientists, we shudder to think of how this scenario maybe played out. Males in many, if not all species of animal life could in effect be chemically neutered. What does this phenomenon called by a Canadian documentary the "disappearing male" mean for our own species 100 years from now if we do not do something to clean up our act?

In the modern world we are literally submerged in EDCs, or Endocrine Disrupting Compounds. These are compounds that have the ability to disrupt the endocrine system, or the hormonal system.` Over 80,000 EDCs are in use in commerce, farming and industry. According to the National Institute of Environmental Health Sciences (NIEHS):

> Pharmaceuticals, fabric treatments, pesticides, fertilizers and other chemicals can disrupt the endocrine systems and can be found in water….Exposure to environmental chemicals, including EDC's in the environment may play an important role in the etiology of diseases…. along with nutrition, infection and stress.

Filtering out EDCs from our public water systems is difficult if not impossible. Water treatment systems in the US were designed to eliminate harmful bacteria, not designed to filter out pharmaceuticals and other chemicals. Consequently, here is a short list of some of the household products that we find in our environment, and more troubling specifically in our water:

- Anti-inflammatories/Analgesics like ibuprofen, naproxen, aspirin
- Seizure medications
- Psychiatric medications and antidepressants
- Cholesterol medications
- Synthetic Hormones including 17 alphaethinylestradiol, 17 beta estradiol, and estrone
- Pesticides, organophosphates, carbamates, pyrethroids, organochlorine
- Blood Pressure medicines like metoprolol and atenolol
- Antibiotics and Antimicrobials including triclosan, sulphonamides, tetracycline
- Diuretics
- Personal Care Products that include insect repellants, preservatives, soaps, sunscreens, fragrances, cosmetics, toothpaste

To point the importance of using pure and safe personal care products, look at a study in Massachusetts involved high school girls, who used cosmetics. Researchers drew and tested the teenage girls blood and urine to assess the known levels of toxic chemicals present in the cosmetics.

Not surprisingly alarmingly high levels of toxic, but commonly used cosmetic chemicals, EDC's, were found in the girl's blood and urine. The researchers stated many of these young women would go on to experience adverse health effects from an ongoing exposure to these chemicals and there would also be those who would struggle with hormonal imbalances and some would even go on to experience infertility. Like in the egg-producing "intersex" fish, EDCs impact the reproductive systems of young girls as well as their entire endocrine system causing problems like polycystic ovarian syndrome, insulin resistant diabetes, obesity, etc.

EDCs: An Explanation for Obesity Epidemic

Many of the EDC's are now considered "Obesogens," or an EDC's that say a child, for example, is exposed to in childhood that causes the child to become obese as an adult. We have seen this with DES (Diethylstilbesterol) exposure. According to Newbold, et al, mice given DES for just 5 days at birth resulted in increased weight in female mice beginning at puberty. This is with absolutely no change in the food intake or exercise of these mice! Photos of their research show a massively obese mouse compared to its sibling not receiving DES for 5 days at birth. There are many chemicals that are now categorized as "obesogens." The obesogen's trigger is a short exposure during early development and leading to obesity later in life.

Without getting too scientific here, what we're talking about is "Epigenetics," the study of "chemical" modifications of DNA and chromatin which are heritable and affect genome function (transcription, replication, recombination), but do not affect the DNA backbone. What does that mean? It means simply that some chemicals that we are exposed to have the ability to modify our DNA and we are able to pass that on to future generations.

Education and Action

What should our response be to all of this? In medicine it might simply mean changing our focus from curing a disease to prevention and intervention strategies to reduce disease incidence. In law it might mean changing the way we currently regulate industrial chemicals. Currently of the 80,000 chemicals used in commerce, only 200 have been tested. Chemicals are generally considered "innocent until proven guilty" in the U.S. That means a potentially harmful chemical could be in the market for 10 plus years before it is discovered to be a problem. It might mean tighter regulatory control over the pharmaceutical industry.

To the average American it is a wake up call to be proactive and educated on health care/medication decisions. We have to take the bull by the horns so to speak. It is our responsibility to control what chemicals our families are exposed to in our foods, homes and environments our families. This means finding and buying good local produce, organic foods, avoiding household chemicals that are harmful, knowing where our meat comes from and how it is produced, filtering our own water, partnering with a personal care company that you know and can trust to use safe ingredients and to be transparent with ingredient policies and green commitments. It means educating oneself and taking action because your future, our future depends upon it.

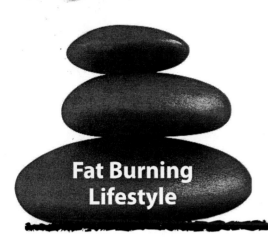

Fat Burning Lifestyle

Using Nutrition and Exercise to Restore Balance

Body fat and estrogen are connected because fat cells produce estrogen. Ever notice that an overweight man will sometimes develop breast tissue? That's the effect of fat cells producing estrogen in his body. Many women at middle age notice they have a thickening waistline and can't seem to get rid of it. A diet with too many carbohydrates can cause an increase in body fat and an increase in circulating estrogen hormone levels. Eliminating processed foods, carbs, the wrong kind of fats and adding exercise to your daily regimen can make a big difference in the way you look and feel. If you are a junk food junkie, drinking more than 2 alcoholic beverages a day, or eating high caloric foods without much fiber and nutritional value, then you are heading in the wrong direction.

The area of obesity and nutrition is very near and dear to our hearts. This area of health and wellness always had been. Our children often shock their teachers with their remarks of why we shouldn't eat too much sugar, or why we avoid MSG and why we eat wild salmon for the Omega 3 fatty acids. Health and nutrition have always been important in the Osborn household. But its imprtance took on a whole new personal meaning one Sunday morning in July of 2006. Chris was getting ready for church, and got a phone call from his sister. She was crying and said, "Dad passed away in his sleep last night." It was like a knife went through his heart. "That can't be!" Chris said. His dad hadn't been sick. He took his medicines for blood pressure and cholesterol. Not to mention, no one in Chris's family dies before they're ninety years old! Chris's grandparents were well into their nineties and still living independently in their own home. His grandfather, a retired country doctor, still drives out to the Amish communities on occasion to check in on them. He's 95 and just went on a cruise to Alaska! There is no way in this world that Chris's Dad could die at a mere 59 years young. The coroner said it was most certainly a heart attack in his sleep, but as this sunk in over the ensuing months, none of it made sense. Then it started to sink in, "He is the only one in our family that was significantly overweight." He was probably 50 pounds overweight. He also had a lot of stress, which causes hormonal imbalances and skyrocketing levels of inflammatory mediators. The discussion of heart disease is sufficient to fill an entire book in and of itself, so we will not elaborate on it here. But since excess fat significantly affects hormone balance, the importance of proper nutrition, weight management and fitness should be adequately discussed now.

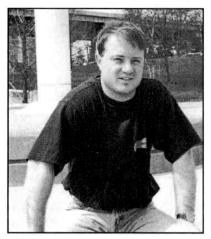

Dr. Chris Osborn – Before

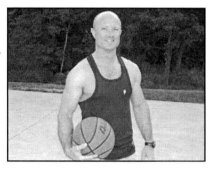

Dr. Chris Osborn – After

Many diseases do not produce any symptoms for years, and then suddenly it seems one day you have high blood pressure, high cholesterol, diabetes and heart disease. These diseases are, in fact, caused by years of poor life style habits. Many people believe they are eating "healthy," but are not. There are a number of books available at the library about this subject so vital to good health and wellness. For example, Dr. David Perlmutter in his book, *The Better Brain Book*, advises us that for better heart, brain and overall health – get the fattening, starchy junk foods off your plate and replace them with real foods such as unprocessed, whole grains loaded with brain-boosting B vitamins and anti-oxidant rich fruits and vegetables. Eliminate the unnecessary sources of sugar that are adding on those extra pounds and wildly accelerating the formation of free radicals. Buy organic produce, meats that are free of added chemicals such as pesticides, growth hormones and antibiotics that can spread inflammation throughout your body.

Exercise

As we stated earlier, hormone imbalance is caused by a variety of factors: diet, lifestyle, medicine and environment. The struggle to find balance in our lives is not easy. However, a comprehensive holistic approach must be taken to achieve balance. If we are going to battle estrogen dominance we must look at nutrition, exercise and body fat. Body fat and estrogen are intricately linked because fat cells produce estrogen. Where there is an excess of body fat, hormone balance is impacted. Due to this fact, the importance of proper nutrition, weight management and exercise needs to be addressed together.

Let us introduce Tara Johnson. Tara earned her Bachelor of Arts degree in Sociology from Providence College in Canada where she was an All-Conference collegiate basketball player. As someone who has dealt with weight issues, Tara Johnson understands the commitment and dedication it takes to make changes in your life, then maintain them and stop the bouts of yoyo dieting and exercise. She works with clients to set goals, develop a plan and modify behaviors to live a full and fit life. She is a certified personal trainer with the American College of Sports Medicine and owner of Get Fit for Life. If you would like to contact Tara see the list of resources in the back of this handbook for contact information.

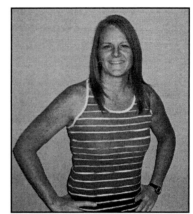

Tara Johnson

This section on exercise by Tara is included to help you develop a "Fat Burning Lifestyle" regimine for being healthy, strong and active. Here's Tara:

Most people today struggle with good nutrition and adequate exercise due to a lack of knowledge, insufficient time and motivation. Why? Typically, the population doesn't get enough sleep leading to getting up "just in time" to go to work and/or get the kids to school. Then too often the domino effect occurs; we rely on caffeine instead of a healthy and nutrient rich breakfast; there is just no time for planning the rest of the day's nutrition and exercise; we grab a quick, fast and usually unhealthy lunch, followed by a afternoon snack, beverage, or both to get through the "mid-day slump;" then we have a large dinner because we have not eaten anything of substance all day. We end the day exhausted, treat ourselves to the nightly snack as our reward for making it through another day. This leaves us full when we awake and the cycle repeats itself again...and again...and again. If only there was a plan, extra time and some motivation?

Imagine that you were able to take a picture of the inside of your body. Right now, you could see the function of your heart, kidneys, lungs, liver, intestines, and colon. Would you look? Would you want to know if you were on the verge of developing high blood pressure, high cholesterol, diabetes and heart disease? What if you already have these diseases? Is medication your long-term plan?

As the doctors have already mentioned, these diseases are, in fact, caused by years of poor lifestyle habits. We neglect the one body we are given and when it begins to fail us, unfortunately, we don't get another.

Physical Fitness

The definition of physical fitness is the freedom from illness, infection, disease and shock and the ability to perform both vocational and recreational tasks without the risk of injury and undo fatigue. What would your life look like if you were the example, a model of physical fitness, according to this definition?

To make the journey manageable, we will break it down into 7 components of physical fitness: Aerobic exercise, Anaerobic exercise, Stretching, Low Body Fat, Realistic Nutrition, Proper Rest, and Stress Management.

Aerobic: Cardiovascular/Respiratory

Aerobic exercise is a must component of a healthy and balanced lifestyle and fitness program. It is necessary for a healthy heart and good respiratory care. Aerobic means in the presence of oxygen and is characterized by any activity that is performed at a low to moderate intensity for more than 60 seconds. This type of exercise allows oxygen to release energy through metabolism and can include running, jogging, walking, swimming and biking. You can use a treadmill, an elliptical, a stationary or recumbent bike or the great outdoors.

During an aerobic workout, the first 12-15 minutes you are burning sugar then you enter into the fat burning stage. An optimal aerobic workout is 45 minutes and no longer than 60 minutes, unless you are an endurance athlete. For this type of exercise you will want to monitor your heart rate to ensure you are in the correct range and stay within this range for the duration of the workout.

To determine your range, use the simple calculation below:

- 220 - Age = Predicted Maximum Heart Rate (PMHR)
- Multiply your PMHR by 85 percent for your maximum base aerobic heart rate.
- Multiply your PMHR by 55 percent for your minimum base aerobic heart rate.

Use these two rates to determine your aerobic heart rate range. It is recommended to stay within this range once warm-up is complete and until cool-down begins.

There are several benefits of aerobic activity: increased cardiovascular function and a decrease in body fat. However, if aerobic activity is your sole type of exercise, keep in mind that there is potential for a decrease in muscle strength, muscle mass, power and speed. To minimize these effects, implement anaerobic exercise into your routine.

Anaerobic: Muscular/Skeletal Strength

Anaerobic by definition means without oxygen. Of course, this does not mean that you exercise without breathing. Put simply, anaerobic exercise is an activity that you complete at a high effort (90-110 percent of your PMHR) and have to stop to recover within 60 - 90 seconds. Your body is producing energy without utilizing oxygen. Anaerobic exercise is vital to build muscle, gain strength, and increase body tone. This type of exercise includes body weight resistance training such as push-ups, pull-ups and squats, free weights or weight machines and interval training such as running sprints.

During an anaerobic workout, your body uses 2 energy pathways. The first is high energy phosphates which are stored in very limited quantities within the muscle cell.

This fuel source will sustain you for the first 5-10 seconds of the activity. Your body will then begin to use the second energy pathway, anaerobic glycolysis, where the body uses the breakdown of glucose for energy. This energy system produces lactic acid and leads to fatigue.

One of the best benefits of anaerobic activity is the after burn or excess post-exercise oxygen consumption (EPOC). EPOC refers to the oxygen consumption the body uses to return to its regular or pre-exercise condition. Remember, we have burned oxygen and high energy phosphates that need to be replenished and have produced lactic acid that the body must remove; not to mention resuming body temperature and blood circulation. The rate and duration of EPOC is dependent on intensity of activity, duration of exercise and continuous versus interval exercise. Studies have shown that the higher the intensity, the longer the duration and the more intervals all increase the rate of EPOC. Some research shows that EPOC after anaerobic activity can last between 12 and 18 hours compared to 2 to 6 hours for aerobic activity. The longer the after burn, the greater the calories burned as you continue on with your day.

There are other benefits to anaerobic exercise: increased cardiovascular function, decreased body fat, increased muscle mass, improved strength, power and speed. One benefit of anaerobic exercise that is overlooked is an increase in aerobic capacity. When you utilize the anaerobic energy pathways, the aerobic pathways benefit also. Unfortunately, there is one catch associated of anaerobic exercise, it requires an aerobic foundation.

So, as we continue the balance theme, know that you must incorporate both aerobic and anaerobic exercise into your life. It is not an either or routine. The goal of any exercise prescription should be to optimize your performance in all aspects of physical activity.

Stretching: Joint Flexibility and Body Elasticity

Stretching may be the most important aspect of physical fitness and the most neglected. Flexibility is defined as the body's ability and freedom to move unrestricted through a joint's range of motion. Elasticity is defined as the body's ability to return to its original shape or condition before it was stretched. Most people don't build this component into their exercise regimen and fail to realize that stretching increases body strength and muscle tone.

There are different ways to stretch, with the most common being static stretch or static flexibility. This is a range of motion that can be achieved by holding a body stretch in a stationary position for a period of time. The primary purpose of this stretch is to relax a muscle and joint group. If you are trying to improve your flexibility, the best time to actively static stretch is at the end of the workout or when the muscle tissue is at a high thermal temperature. The best way to achieve the benefits of static stretching is to hold the stretch for a minimum of 20 to 30 seconds, but no longer than 60 seconds, as the benefits will not increase.

Prior to an exercise or stretching routine beginning, a warm-up lasting at least 5 minutes should be implemented. This warm-up allows the muscle tissue's temperature and blood flow to increase. Including a warm-up pre-exercise or stretch will greatly reduce the risk of injury. The warm-up can include low intensity aerobic exercise such as walking or biking or a low intensity dynamic exercise such as skipping or jumping jacks.

If you are looking for a simple and effective exercise program, we recommend a 4-day split. This will require setting aside a minimum of 4 days per week for exercise. Here is how is breaks down:

- 4 days of anaerobic or strength training followed by aerobic or cardio training. It is important to complete your strength training before you perform any cardio so you can use the energy stored in your muscles to lift the heaviest weight possible. The duration of each will be dependent on how much time you have available, but should include no more than 50 percent of your time performing cardio training. Remember to spend a minimum of 5 minutes warming up before starting a workout.
- You will have one rest day or an optional cardio training day in the middle of the 4-day split.
- You will have a second rest day or an optional leisure activity that needs to last a minimum of 30 minutes. This can include mowing the grass, playing basketball with your kids, going for a walk, etc.

- You will then set aside one day to completely rest and give your body time to rejuvenate.
- The following layout is to be used as a guide.

	Sun	Mon	Tue	Wed	Thu	Fri	Sat
Anaerobic	OFF	Strength - Upper body	Strength - Lower body	Rest	Strength - Upper body	Strength - Lower body	Rest
Aerobic	OFF	(Optional)	(Optional)	30-60 min (Optional)	(Optional)	(Optional)	30 min - Leisure activity (Optional)
Stretching	OFF	5 min	5 min	5 min	5 min	5 min	5 min

Low Body Fat

As was stated in the introduction to this section, body fat and estrogen are intricately connected because fat cells produce estrogen. To achieve a proper hormone balance and great overall health, we must maintain our ideal weight and body fat percentage. Along with being a trigger for hormone imbalance, excess body fat is now recognized as a primary risk factor for coronary heart disease, cancer, diabetes, and autoimmune disorders by the American College of Sports Medicine.

• Description	• Women	• Men
• Essential fat	• 10–13%	• 2–5%
• Athletes	• 14–20%	• 6–13%
• Fitness	• 21–24%	• 14–17%
• Average	• 25–31%	• 18–24%
• Obese	• 32%+	• 25%+

To be clear, this section is titled "Low Body Fat", not "No Body Fat". Body fat serves several vital functions.

1. Insulation - we need fat to keep us warm
2. Cushion - we need fat as a layer of protection
3. Fuel - we need fat to give us energy to move and exercise
4. Transportation - we need fat to move vitamins and minerals throughout our body

Bioidentical Hormone Handbook: Restoring Balance Through BHRT, Detox, Nutrition and Exercise

With that said, how much fat is enough? The American Council on Exercise provides the following chart for reference.

One thing to consider when determining where you should be on this chart is body type or somatotype. There are 3 different somatotypes: Ectomorph, Endomorph and Mesomorph. Whether you are male or female, having an understanding of your body type will help clarify where you should fall in the range of body fat percentage.

- Ectomorph - characterized by smaller, lengthy bones and a struggle to add muscle mass
- Endomorph - characterized by a pear shape frame, larger bone structure and a higher total body mass
- Mesomorph - characterized by medium sized bones, athletic structure and a significant amount of lean

Knowing your body type can provide greater understanding of what your ideal body fat should be. For example, if you are a female Ectomorph, your body fat could be between 16-21 percent to be healthy compared to a female Endomorph who would still be considered healthy if her body fat fell between 21-25 percent.

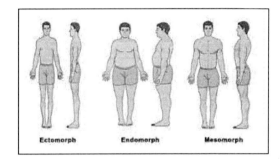

It can be difficult and expensive to get an exact measurement of your body fat percentage. There are many methods available, but most are inaccurate and unreliable. The gold standard is underwater weighing where your weight is compared while immersed in water to your weight on dry land. However, this can be very costly and not easily accessible. Using skin-fold calipers and electrical impedance devices are highly variable and almost of no use because of operator error, liquid intake prior to measurement and the female's cycle.

One method for determining body fat is to use the Body Mass Index (BMI). This chart, which was invented between 1830 and 1850, uses your current height and weight to assess an individual's body weight from what is normal or desirable for a person of his or her height. The BMI does provide ranges from severely underweight to 3 levels of obesity, however everyone should remember that these are only statistical categories that should be viewed as a guide. You can find a copy of the Body Mass Index or a BMI calculator online.

If you need to lose weight, you must create a caloric deficit, meaning that you expend more energy (calories) than you are bringing in. One pound of body mass is equal to 3500 calories, so to lose 1 pound per week, you must create a caloric deficit of 500 calories per day. We highly recommend utilizing a food journal to record each calorie that is taken in. Most people have no idea how much food they are actually eating. If you are going to be successful at creating a deficit you must know what you are taking in. There are many smart phone applications and websites that make this task much easier. For most people, disciplining themselves to 1400-1600 calories per day will result in consistent and long-term weight loss. Typically, you will want to lose 1-1.5 pounds per week. This will ensure that your body is adapting to long-term change and increases your odds of sticking with it.

Another vital key to health is hydration. You must be drinking half of your body weight in ounces of water everyday. For example, if you currently weigh 150 pounds, you will need to drink 75 ounces of water per day. There is 70 percent water consistency in our bodies and most of us live in a constant state of dehydration. Water hydrates your body and provides the medium for proper digestion, nerve firing and body communication. Besides, fat is not soluble in water, so water will push fat through cell walls, into the liver and kidneys for the process of excretion. Water is a must for overall health!

Proper Rest

Our bodies need rest in order to function at a high level during the hours we are required to be awake. Allan Holson, director of the Laboratory of Neurophysiology at Harvard states, "Consistent, high quality sleep is where our bodies and our minds recover, restore and grow from all of the events and circumstances of our lives that occurred the day before." Your body is doing amazing things while you sleep and for overall health, we must allow time for proper rest.

In his book *The Seven Pillars of Health*, Dr. Don Colbert gives five reasons why sleep and rest are so important for physical fitness and wellness.

- Sleep regulates the release of important hormones, such as Human Growth Hormone, or HGH, which regulates muscle mass and helps control fat and leptin, which directly influences appetite and weight control.
- Sleep slows the aging process.
- Sleep boosts your autoimmune system by releasing white blood cells during sleep that destroy viruses and bacteria.
- Sleep improves brain function.
- Sleep reduces cortisol levels raised by excessive stress. High cortisol levels are associated with an excess of body fat.

So, with all those benefits happening while you rest, it is recommended that you get 7 to 9 hours of sleep per night.

Stress Management

As was just stated, high cortisol levels are associated with excess body fat and are raised by excessive stress. Stress is defined by Hans Sayle as any stimulus that places an adaptive demand of the systems of the mind and body. By this definition, stress is not inherently bad and can be something that is productive for us. However, our bodies begin to break down when the level of stress goes beyond our capabilities and limits. Fortunately, physical fitness increases your metabolic rate and burns off the harmful effects of stress, both emotionally and physiologically, while at the same time naturally contributing to hormone balance.

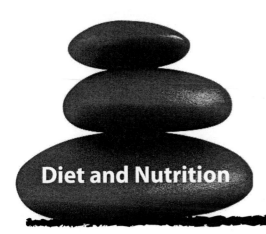

Diet and Nutrition

"Health is not valued until sickness comes."
— Dr. Thomas Fuller

Good nutrition is vital to good health. Giving the body what it needs and then keeping away from foods that are difficult to digest or just plain not good for us, like corn syrup, sugar, and simple carbs, will work to bring about a higher level of body efficiency and energy. In selecting the elements and the "how-to" for this important section, we sought the able guidance of Barbara Beaty, who has her Ph.D. in nutritional counseling.

Along with Dr. Beaty and others, we have worked to bring this simple eating plan to you to assist you in reforming your food selections and food quantities throughout each day for optimum health results.

Many people don't realize that fatigue, foggy thinking, poor sleep, excess weight (especially around the stomach, hips and thighs) and even aging skin indicate nutritional deficiencies that can be reversed. Adopting a healthier lifestyle for you and your family can be easy to talk about, but difficult to get started without a plan. The following 30 Days to Feeling Fit plan is simple to follow and therefore, simple to complete. The plan focuses on five key areas of fitness:

30 Days to Feeling Fit

1. Eat Clean
2. Increase Nutrient Intake
3. Eliminate Allergenic and Addictive Foods
4. Balance Blood Sugar
5. Detox: Support Elimination Organs

1. Eat Clean

Fitness requires eating organic whole foods, free of gluten, preservatives, additives, pesticides, hormones, antibiotics, artificial colors and flavors, and all other toxins, because food is either fuel or poison. Simply put, anything that can't be used as energy in the body is a toxin. Organic fruits and vegetables contain up to 40 percent more antioxidants than those conventionally grown. This plan will help you learn how to fuel your body for optimal health by eating clean, close to nature and TOXIN FREE!

2. Increase Nutrient Intake

Due to the overabundance of pre-packaged and fast food, many people today are overweight yet malnourished. They carry toxic fat while their bodies are starving for real nutrition. This condition can be reversed by eating whole foods and supplementing with nutrients to fill in possible deficiencies created by mineral deficient farm soils.

3. Eliminate Allergenic and Addictive Foods

Many people experience symptoms of premature aging or poor health and have no idea that the solution may be as simple as removing possible food allergens. This

Candida (Yeast) Overgrowth

Candida overgrowth in your body will cause you to suffer from sugar cravings. Candida yeast loves sugar just as much as you do, and it's love of this empty, non-nutritional food causes you to want it more.

- *According to a study done at Rice University, "70 percent of American's are living daily with an overgrowth of yeast and bacteria."*

- *Signs of yeast overgrowth include: nasal congestion and discharge, nasal itching, blisters in the mouth, sore or dry throat, abdominal pain, belching, bloating, heartburn, constipation, diarrhea, rectal burning or itching, vaginal discharge, vaginal itching or burning, worsening symptoms of PMS, prostatitis, impotence, frequent urination, burning on urination, bladder infections.*

- *Candida yeast is known to feed on dairy, gluten, wheat, sugar, caffeine and alcohol. Eliminating these repopulate the intestines with friendly bacteria which help the body fight off the Candida, and strengthen the immune system.*

plan includes removing possible allergenic foods like gluten, dairy, soy and processed sugars. If you cringe at the thought of removing a certain food, chances are you are allergic to it. Generally speaking, the food you crave is the food that is killing you.

Gluten is a family of proteins found in grains. They are thick and gooey and make things stick together when baked, instead of falling apart. It is estimated that 50 percent of the population has difficulty breaking down gluten in their intestines.

When the immune system recognizes gluten in the gut as a "foreign protein," it attacks and damages the intestinal wall, which in turn causes the intestines to swell with water creating bloating and/or a "pot belly." Eventually, the intestinal wall thins to the point that it starts absorbing things that should have been blocked causing an array of problems including:

> **Allergies:** The tips of the villi in the intestines produce the enzyme that digests the lactose in milk. Since they're the first to go, the very first symptom of gluten intolerance you see may be a "milk allergy" that manifests itself as a stuffy nose and post-nasal drip that occurs whenever you consume dairy products.

> **Immune Function:** The constant load on the immune system as it fights off foreign proteins in the digestive tract impairs its ability to do its job elsewhere. Meanwhile, clogged sinuses and unhealthy intestinal walls create a perfect home for harmful bacteria to multiply.

> **Adrenal Function:** The constant adrenal load created by chronic inflammation of the intestines eventually leads to adrenal insufficiency or even adrenal exhaustion. As the adrenals become impaired, many other symptoms manifest themselves, including allergies, slow weight gain and a loss of energy.

Dairy

Despite the widespread notion that milk is healthy, drinking pasteurized milk is frequently associated with a *worsening* of health. Sally Fallon of the Weston Price Foundation states, *"Pasteurization destroys enzymes, diminishes vitamin content, denatures fragile milk proteins, destroys vitamin B12 and vitamin B6, kills beneficial bacteria, promotes pathogens and is associated with allergies."* Only 30 percent of the calcium in a cup of milk gets absorbed, you would get twice as much calcium from a cup of broccoli. Many green leafy vegetables are loaded with calcium.

Soy

Phytoestrogens in soy can mimic the effects of the female hormone estrogen. These phytoestrogens have been found to have adverse effects on various human tissues. Drinking two glasses of soy milk daily for one month has enough of the chemical to alter a woman's menstrual cycle. Note: Soy Lecithin does not have the same effect and is safe for those sensitive to soy.

Refined Sugar

Refined sugar has been stripped of all nutrients and drains and leaches the body of precious vitamins and minerals. Sugar taken every day produces a continuously acidic condition which affects every organ in the body. Initially sugar is stored in the liver. A daily intake of refined sugar makes the liver expand like a balloon. When the liver is filled to its maximum capacity, the excess sugar is returned to the blood in the form of fatty acids. These are stored (and seen) in the most inactive areas: the belly, the buttocks, and the thighs. In contrast unrefined sugar like cane sugar contains minerals the body needs.

> Dr. Michael McCann, MD, physician and researcher, states, "Probiotics will be to medicine in the twenty-first century as antibiotics and microbiology were in the twentieth century."

4. Balanced Blood Sugar

30 Days to Feeling Fit encourages eating low on the glycemic index for many reasons. The high, moderate and low "glycemic index" is a measure of how a given food affects blood-sugar levels, with each food being assigned a numbered rating. The lower the rating, the more gradual the infusion of sugars into the bloodstream and the more balanced the blood sugar.

High glycemic meals cause you to feel hungry soon after you eat. Eating low glycemic meals reduces hunger cravings. When blood sugar goes up in response to a high glycemic meal a process called "glycation" takes place, which promotes thinning of the skin and wrinkles. It's not just candy bars and cupcakes that elevate blood sugar. Pasta, bread, potatoes, white rice and other high glycemic fruits are also responsible.

5. Detox: Support Elimination Organs

As you repair fitness and health through good diet and nutrition, it would be incomplete if it did not support the body's five elimination pathways: the liver, kidneys, intestines and your largest detoxifying organ, your skin. It is nearly impossible to avoid the toxins we come in contact with on a daily basis. If toxins enter your body faster than they are removed, you will experience signs of toxicity. If, on the other hand, you give your body the support it needs to eliminate these toxins, it will perform optimally.

Liver, Kidney, and Intestinal Support

We wouldn't think about going a day without brushing our teeth, let alone years and years. Because we can't see our liver, kidneys, and intestines we forget the important role they play in detoxification. The liver has over 500 functions and the kidneys filter 200 quarts of blood per day. You can hold 5-25 pounds of waste in your large intestine (colon). All elimination organs need a "tune up" and proper maintenance.

A good detox tea assists the daily cleansing of the liver and kidneys by helping the body to filter and clear toxins. This in turn regulates cholesterol, balances blood sugar and promotes weight loss. Many are unaware that liver dysfunction is more closely related to obesity than any other single factor. An overburdened liver is one of the reasons people plateau during weight loss.

Also helpful is a detox regimine to help cleanse and detoxify the system and support the liver, kidneys, and gastrointestinal (GI) tract. This assists with the gentle elimination of heavy metals and other environmental toxins.

Skin Support

Soaking 30 minutes in a bath of seawater or mineral salts literally draws toxins and heavy metals through the pores of the skin. Aches and pains will melt away and you'll find yourself sleeping better at night. For thousands of years people have enjoyed the healing benefits of seawater.

Your skin is your largest detoxifying organ. It is designed to both absorb nutrients and release toxins. Many people are very careful about what they put in their mouth but don't consider the toxins they are putting on their skin every day. It takes only 26 seconds for the toxic ingredients in skincare to find their way into every organ of your body.

Concluding Remarks

After years as family practitioners and seeing countless patients, we know good health is a work. It takes a clear decision by each of us to take charge of our own health position. We are delighted to offer you this handbook with just enough details so you can get in the driver's seat to maintain or regain health, maybe for the first time. Following the simple steps in this handbook can make a huge difference in your life, in the health of your family, and has the potential to positively impact the world around you.

We have learned that traditional medicine doesn't always have all the answers, and sometimes the answers are just downright wrong. If we had followed the advice of traditional medicine, Deanna would have had a hysterectomy five years ago and probably be on multiple medications now. We chose a different path that led her to health. Deanna often says that she feels better now than she did even as a teenager! There are so many men and women out there that can learn from our experience and hopefully get back on track.

Why do you need to be in charge of your health? In today's busy medical practices, doctors simply don't have time to educate patients about health and/or diseases and their treatments. This handbook is intended to begin your health learning curve, so you can become an active participant, along with your doctor, in improving your health position. Health requires you to know your body better than anyone else. If you are certain something is just not right, then please, get "outside the traditional treatment box" and take time to read and research, to get a better understanding, especially to learn what you can do.

The foundation of the guidance we offer is to first balance your hormones, which means clear, concise messages are being delivered to all your body systems; then cleaning up those body systems with a thorough, yet gentle, detoxing; add a good at home exercise regimen, so you too can be fit without expensive gym fees. This coupled with proper nutrition and nutritional supplements provides a winning combination for health.

The material offered here is simple to understand, but so many of you may feel like you have so much to learn. So take your time. All who have started the journey to health have, at times, been overwhelmed. Start with one of the 4 sections and familiarize yourself with it. Master it, if you like, and then move to the next section. We believe it will take 30 days to make a transition from where you are to be solidly on the track to good health, energy and vitality.

Health and feeling fit is an exciting prospect and significant improvement is within reach. You can begin to see a difference right away. This initial success helps give us the heart needed to stay the course. Give us 30 days and we will show you how quickly changes can be made in your health.

The temptations are great and it is easier to let go and let others take responsibility for preventing disease, instead of maintaining our own health. Get outside the disease box that has us only seeking a remedy or treatment when a health issue arises and presses against us.

Finally, you can make a difference in the world around you. By becoming aware of the adverse effects that synthetic hormones are having on our environment. To ignore this issue, which is largely what our government has done, is ethically wrong and dangerous. Imagine our world 100 years into the future, are men going to be exposed to such high quantities of estrogen that they are no longer able to reproduce just as the male fish in the Potomac River have been feminized to the point that 30 percent of the male fish are able to produce eggs? If this comes about, we can expect changes for the human species as well.

We invite you to use this handbook to get ahead of disease and dysfunction and live life to its fullest. Together we can make a difference for ourselves, our children, and our children's children, by each one of us becoming healthier, developing water treatment systems that filter out pharmaceuticals, and by insisting that meat produced for human consumption does not contain growth hormones. It takes you to make a difference in your life and it takes only one person to make a huge difference in the larger world.

~*Chris and Deanna*

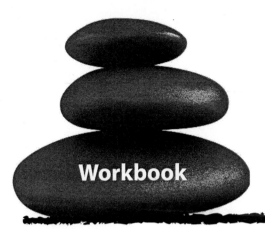

Workbook

Let's Get Started: Food Focus

Eliminate

- Dairy
- Gluten
- Soy
- Peanut Butter
- Table Sugar, Honey, Maple Syrup and Artificial Sweeteners
- Coffee
- Alcohol
- All Fruit EXCEPT Limes, Lemons, Green Apples and Berries
- Pork
- Farm Raised Fish
- Non Cage-Free Eggs
- Non Free-Range Chicken
- All Beef, other than grass fed
- White Potatoes
- Corn
- Nitrites
- MSG
- Vinegar

Include

- Rice, Almond and Coconut Milk
- Brown Rice Millet
- Raw Almonds
- Legumes
- Stevia, Xylitol
- Green and Herb Teas
- Non Starchy Vegetables
- Organic Green Apples and Berries
- Cage-Free Eggs
- Wild Cold Water Fish *(due to possible mercury contamination limit fish to 1x per week)*
- Free-Range Chicken and Turkey
- Grass Fed Beef (1x per week)
- Almond Butter
- Sweet Potatoes, Yams, Turnips
- Avocado
- Olive Oil, Coconut Oil, Flaxseed Oil

The Balanced Eating Circle

When planning your meals think of how you would place food on a plate.

Portion Size Guide

1/2	of the plate = Non-Starchy Vegetables
1/4	of the plate = Lean Protein (fist size) or Protein Shake
3/16	of the plate = High Fiber Carbohydrates and Low Glycemic Fruits*
1/16	of the plate = Healthy Fats

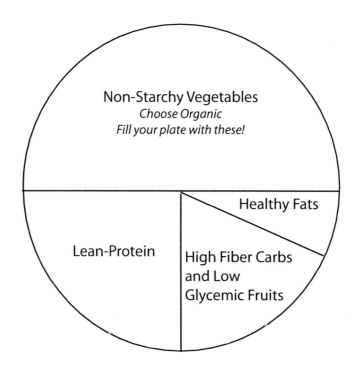

* Moderate and High Glycemic Fruits allowed after workouts or if not trying to lose additional weight

Clean Food Choices

LEAN PROTEIN	Vegan Protein Shake; lean chicken; lean turkey; wild cold water fish (salmon, halibut, cod, mackerel, sardines); grass-fed, lean red meats (1x per week); lamb; game; cage-free and organic eggs
HEALTHY FATS	Raw nuts, seeds (no peanuts), macadamia nuts, freshly ground flaxseed, olive oil, olives, flaxseed oil, cod liver oil, avocado, coconut milk, almond milk, almond butter
HIGH FIBER CARBS	Squash (acorn, butternut, winter), artichokes, leeks, lima beans, okra, pumpkin, sweet potato or yam, turnips, legumes (black lentils, adzuki beans, cow peas, chick peas, french beans, kidney beans, lentils, mung beans, navy beans, pinto beans, split peas, white beans, yellow beans), brown rice, quinoa, hummus, millet
FRUIT GLYCEMIC INDEX	**Low GI:** Blackberries, blueberries, boysenberries, elderberries, raspberries, strawberries, sour green apple **Moderate GI:** Cherries, pears, apricots, melons, oranges, peaches, plums, grapefruit, pitted prunes, apples, avocados, kiwi, lemons, limes, nectarines, tangerines, passion fruit, persimmons, pomegranates **High GI:** (avoid during weight loss except after a workout) Bananas, pineapples, grapes, watermelon, mango, papaya
NON- STARCHY VEGETABLES	Arugula, asparagus, bamboo shoots, bean sprouts, beet greens, bell peppers, broad beans, broccoli, brussel sprouts, cabbage, cassava, carrots, cauliflower, celery, chayote fruit, chicory, chives, collard greens, cucumber, jicama (raw), jalapeño peppers, kale, kohlrabi, lettuce, mushrooms, mustard greens, onions, parsley, radishes, eggplant, endive, fennel, garlic, ginger root, green beans, hearts of palm, radicchio, snap beans, snow peas, shallots, spinach, spaghetti squash, summer squash, swiss chard, tomatoes, turnip greens, watercress

Helpful Notes

Most supermarkets and grocery stores now have healthier food choices, organic brands and a designated aisle just for health food. Do not feel like you need a Health Food Store to find the food/ingredients you need to start your program. However, if you do have a local health food store, Whole Foods Market or Trader Joe's nearby, it would be great to start your shopping there.

If you are going to a health food store to shop for the first time, make sure you have time to look around and plan on asking for help. Everyone that works in these stores is ready to help and is usually very knowledgeable.

When you make your shopping list for the first week, start with the foods on the Clean Food Choices list that you already like. Ease into the program on food you are familiar with and enjoy eating. You WILL need to switch to cage free proteins, grass fed beef, organic high fiber carbohydrates, fruits and vegetables whenever possible. This way we are not ingesting toxins with the foods we eat.

Follow the meal plan on page 66 when making your list; this makes it easier when going to the store the first time. A list keeps you on track, helps you remember everything you need and keeps you from feeling lost. This way if you need to ask for something, you know what it is and can ask for it by name.

Buy Organic
There is usually an organic alternative to everything, just do your homework. If you want, you can shop online first so you know what is available before you ever step foot inside the store.

Clean Food Shopping Overview

Lean Proteins
Organic cage-free, hormone-free and free-range meats are found in meat markets, health food stores or sometimes even at COSTCO. Only buy organic grass-fed beef and organic chicken. As for fish, purchase wild (never farmed) fresh or canned (in water).

Free Range eggs come from hens that are allowed to grow and peck the ground. They are fed grain, seeds, and greens that contain a higher level of essential fatty acids than non-free range hens. Free range hens do not eat feed that has been treated with antibiotics and other chemicals.

Healthy Fats

Use Extra Virgin Olive Oil (EVOO) in salad dressings and for low heat sautéing. Use Coconut Oil for high heat sautéing. Olive oil turns rancid (becomes toxic) under medium high heat, whereas Coconut Oil maintains its integrity when heated. Coconut oil is solid at room temperature. It is most often sold in jars alongside all the standard bottled oils. Avoid high-oleic safflower, corn and canola oils as they are highly processed. Enjoy small servings of avocado, coconut milk, olives, raw nuts and seeds.

High Fiber Carbohydrates

DRY PACKAGED Legumes and grains such as brown rice are often packaged and sold in ethnic or health food sections of grocery stores. Trader Joe's even has vacuum-sealed packaged cooked brown rice (add diced veggies and EVOO for a delicious grain salad).

FROZEN Look for cooked squash, artichoke hearts, lima beans and other vegetables.

CANNED Watch out for high sodium. Read labels and compare beans, artichoke hearts (in water), organic soups and organic broths.

REFRIGERATED hummus, salsa, rice tortillas, cooked lentils, grain salads and pesto.

Why Grass Fed Beef?

Grass-fed beef is naturally leaner than grain-fed beef. The Omega 3 content in beef that feed on grass is 7 percent of the total fat content, compared to 1 percent in grain-only fed beef.

Grass-fed beef has the recommended ratio of omega 6 to omega 3 fats (3:1).

Grass-fed beef is loaded with other natural minerals and vitamins, plus it's a great source of CLA (conjugated linoleic acid) a fat that reduces the risk of cancer, obesity, diabetes and a number of immune disorders.

Meat production of non- grass fed beef includes hormones, tranquilizers, pesticides and antibiotics (40 percent of all the antibiotics produced in the United States are fed to animals). We eat those animals and those chemicals become a part of us. The overuse of antibiotics in our food production is one of the reasons antibiotic resistant diseases are on the rise.

Meal Plan

Pick out your favorite recipes using clean foods and plan your meals for the week. Substitute 1-2 protein shakes per day for ANY meal. Enjoy a variety of green leafy veggies with every meal.

	Breakfast	Lunch	Dinner
Day 1			
Day 2			
Day 3			
Day 4			
Day 5			
Day 6			
Day 7			

Shopping List

Refer to your weekly meal plan and make your clean and whole food shopping list. Use coconut oil for sautéing (remains healthy when heated). Use EVOO for raw food and dressings.

Lean Protein	
Healthy Fats	
High Fiber Carbs	
Non Starchy Vegetables	
Supplements and Dietary Aids	

7 Simple Steps to Get Started

1. Day One
   - Weigh yourself and record your waist measurements (at belly button and 2" below belly button)

2. Go shopping and get prepared
   - Get rid of all the temptations in your cabinets and fill your kitchen with healthy choices.
   - Let your friends and family know what you are doing so they can support you for the 30 days!

3. Water is your best friend
   - Drink at least six 8 ounce glasses of water per day. If you get hungry drink between meals.

4. Eat every 4 hours
   - No snacking except low-cal energy drink supplement, 1 teaspoon of almond butter or small handful of almonds.
   - An exception is the "after workout recovery" shake to nourish your muscles. If having an after workout shake, your next meal is when you feel hungry.
   - Do not go more than 6 hours without having a meal

5. Do not obsess!
   - Don't obsess over weight.
   - Only weigh yourself 1 time per week - NOT EVERYDAY!
   - Have only healthy cleansing foods in your home/office.

6. Do not over eat when eating meals.
   - Fill your plate with veggies. Add fist size protein and grains.
   - NO SECOND SERVINGS! Take your time eating.
   - Chew your food.

7. Track your success.
   - Write a food journal daily and keep a personal journal on how you feel each day.
   - Keep track of your weight loss once a week.
   - Try on clothes that were tight in the past.

Q + A

I am hungry.
- Make sure you are getting a fist size of protein at every meal.
- If your protein source is a shake, make sure you eat an abundance of non-starchy vegetables.
- Make sure you are drinking enough water
- Drink your snacks – have some water with fiber, Detox Tea or vegetable broth

I am not losing weight.
- Some people will not lose any weight until the third week – Stay with it!
- Be sure you are not loading up calories in your shakes.
- Eat plenty of non-starchy vegetables

Why do I feel bloated after my shakes?
- Use a digestive aid in your shakes
- Reduce the amount of fiber you are supplementing

I am losing weight and don't want to.
- Add more calories and fat to your shakes
- Eat any fruit you desire
- Add a starchy carbohydrate to your meals (brown rice).
- Put an extra scoop of protein in your shakes

I am constipated.
- Make sure you are drinking enough water throughout the day at least eight 8 ounce glasses.
- Make sure you are getting enough vegetables
- Add ground flax seed and selium
- Try an herbal colon cleanse

The process of detoxifying can make you feel sluggish, physically and mentally. It's not unusual to feel worse before you feel better. The nutrition and digestive support you will receive from multivitamins, minerals, probitoics and enzymes will assist your body in eliminating toxins at a more rapid rate.

A Sample Day

Wake-up
Cup of Detox Tea

Breakfast
Protein shake made with coconut, rice or almond milk. Add fresh or frozen berries or veggies and 1 teaspoon of almond butter
Add ½ to 1 Scoop Fiber
Take nutritional supplements/multivitamins and minerals

Snack (optional)
Energy drink, if you need something else, have a small handful of raw nuts, seeds or a teaspoon of almond butter

Lunch (4 hours after breakfast)
A fist size of lean protein, non-starchy veggies, brown rice or other high fiber carbohydrates, a small amount of healthy fat or protein shake prepared as above

Snack (see above)

Dinner – 4 hours after lunch
Fist size lean protein, non-starchy veggies, brown rice or other high fiber carb, small amount of healthy fat

DO NOT EAT AFTER 7PM – HAVE A CUP OF DETOX TEA AFTER DINNER

Recovery Shake
If you workout intensely for an hour or more, make sure you have a recovery shake within 30 minutes of completing your workout. Your next meal will be within 4 hours or when you become hungry. The recovery shake is in addition to your healthy meal plan.

Shake Recipes:

The Basics of How to Make a Shake
- 2 Scoops Protein Shake (Chocolate, Vanilla or both)
- ½ to 1 scoop Fiber
- Ice (optional)
- ¼ cup berries (optional)
- Or
- ¼ cup spinach or squash (optional)
- Mix with your choice of the following liquids:
  1 cup water
  ½-1 cup coconut milk, rice milk or unsweetened almond milk
- Add 1 serving of fat:
  1 tsp. almond, walnut, flax or coconut oil (no peanut butter)
  ¼ cup coconut milk or coconut water
  1 TBS ground flax
  1 TBS nuts
  ¼ avocado
  Feel free to experiment with the consistency and ingredients in your shakes to your liking. More ice for thicker shakes.

Helpful Hints for Shakes
- Magic Bullet works great to blend shakes. Sold at Bed, Bath and Beyond or Costco.
- Freeze fresh fruit and veggies for future.
- Add fresh spinach to shakes (won't taste it!)

Chocolate Almond Shake (Version 1)
- 2 Scoops chocolate protein powder
- 1 T almond butter, ice, water or almonds

Chocolate Almond Shake (Version 2)
- 2 Scoops chocolate protein powder
- 1 scoop fiber
- 1 tablespoon almond butter
- Water
- Ice

Chocolate Berry Shake
2 Scoops chocolate protein powder, ¼ cup strawberries, fiber, ice, water

Chocolate Shake
2 Scoops chocolate protein powder, 1 scoop Fiber, water, ice

Chocolate Strawberry Shake
1 scoop chocolate protein shake
1 scoop Fiber
Fresh organic strawberries to taste
Water
Ice

Chocolate Vanilla Combo Shake
1 scoop chocolate protein powder
1 scoop vanilla protein powder
1 scoop fiber
Water and ice

Benefits of Using Coconut Milk in Protein Shakes

Helps the body maintain blood sugar levels
Poor glucose tolerance may mean a deficiency of manganese in the body. Coconut milk is an excellent source of this essential mineral.

Keeps blood vessels and skin elastic and flexible
The mineral copper is critically important for many bodily functions.
Together with vitamin C, it helps keep blood vessels and skin elastic and flexible.

Assists in Weight Control
Medium chain fatty acids in the coconut milk (MCTs) are used in the body for energy, as opposed to long chained fatty acids ((LDTs), that are stored as fat. Medium chain fatty acids create "thermo genesis" in the body which increases metabolism and burns energy.

To find a store near you that carries fresh coconut milk in the refrigerator section go to: nhttp://sodeliciousdairyfree.com/locations/store_locator.php

---

Chocolate Vanilla Chai Shake
1 scoop each of chocolate and vanilla protein powder, almond milk, pumpkin pie spice

Pumpkin Pie Shake
2 scoops vanilla protein powder, 4 ozs pumpkin puree, 1 cup almond milk, pumpkin pie spice, stevia, 1T pecans, fiber

Savory Shake
Heat any veggies (broccoli, zucchini, cauliflower, squash). Puree. Add protein powder, fiber, cooked grain, whole grain milk or broth. Blend.

Vanilla Berry Shake
2 scoops vanilla protein powder, ¼ cup frozen mixed berries, fiber, ice, water

Vanilla Fruit Smoothie
1 scoop vanilla protein powder
1 scoop fiber
Add mixed berry blend to taste
Fresh strawberries
Water and ice

The Importance of Post-Workout Nutrition: Recovery Secrets
By Lanty O'Connor

Refueling the muscles after a workout is essential for any athlete looking to maximize gains and prepare for the next workout. If your muscles are not receiving the correct macronutrients, in the correct amounts, at the correct time, you are losing out on better performance. My experience is that most people don't properly refuel after a workout. Usually one (if not more) of three things happens:

- *Nothing is consumed after a workout*
- *The wrong things are consumed after a workout*
- *The timing of the recovery is incorrect*

So here's what you need to know about post-workout nutrition:

First, let's briefly discuss some exercise physiology. Glycogen is a major fuel source during a workout. Glycogen is stored in the muscles and in the liver. The more highly trained an individual is, the more glycogen is stored in the muscles. After a work-out, the glycogen reserves are highly depleted. Additionally, protein breakdown is also high after a workout. In a 1980 article it was discovered that protein is used for fuel at a much higher rate than is generally assumed. This means that after a workout, the body is in a depleted, catabolic state.

So how do we deal with this state of depletion and catabolism? The answer is insulin. Insulin is the master recovery hormone. High-glycemic index carbohydrates will maximally stimulate insulin to begin the process of refueling the muscles.

The timing of what you consume after a workout is essential. We know that glycogen levels are low and protein breakdown is high after a workout. It has been demonstrated that there is a window of 30 minutes after exercise that is optimal for refueling. During that time period, the body is most able to recover. Ingestion of carbohydrates during the 30 minute window maximally increases insulin levels which promotes glycogen restoration. Additionally, increasing levels of insulin after exercise increases an optimal hormonal environment and can serve as a potent stimulator of protein synthesis.

Recommended 30 Days to Fit Products

Progesterone – Transdermal

Use a natural balancing cream made without mineral oil, free of colors and fragrance, in an air and light tight container that delivers 20 mg of USP bioidentical progesterone.

It is recommended to use ¼ tsp. (1 pump) to ½ tsp. per day. One pump should be applied in the evening; two pumps should be divided, one in the morning, one in the evening. Apply cream to the soft tissues, such as the chest, inner arms, neck, face, palms of the hands, and soles of the feet. It is recommended to rotate applications to a different soft tissue with each usage.

Detox

Fiber added to your daily food intake is important to soothe the colon and helps you to feel satisfied longer and supports balanced blood. Just twelve grams of fiber accounts for nearly half of the recommended daily amount and a flavorless blend of soluble fiber, which is largely undetectable, can be added to all foods and beverages, including protein shakes.

Herbal Detox Tea
Herbal tea is more than a beverage; some can be used as a remedy and for support of the liver and proper body function, as well as a daily "clean up." A tea with the following herbs can be very useful: Milk Thistle, (fruit), Peppermint, (leaf), Dandelion (root), Sweet Fennel (fruit), Elder (flower), Parsley (leaf), Walnut (leaf), Uva Ursi (leaf), Licorice (root).

A 7 - 14 Day Detox Body Cleanse
Periodically, seasonally or monthly, cleansing the body of cellular waste and heavy metals while supporting the detoxifying organs and avenues – the liver, the skin, the lungs, and the colon is an important health maintenance measure as well preparing the body for weight loss. Just eat clean, no sugar, alcohol, or simple carbs, just vegetables, fruit and lean meats along with a detox cleanse.

Detox Soak

Bath treatments have been used for centuries for assisting the skin, the largest external detoxing organ, in ridding the body of toxins is helpful.

Nutrition and Supplements

Digestive Aid with digestive enzymes, prebiotics and a probiotic to support the intestinal wall often damaged by allergenic foods. Probiotics scrub away yeast overgrowth in the lower GI and reestablish friendly bacteria.

Protein Shakes that are vegan, made without dairy or soy, and free of gluten, no trans fats, artificial sweeteners, flavors or colors, are preferable. Drinking meals is easier on digestion and allows our body to have energy for detoxification and is useful as a quick and easy recovery shake after a workout.

Energy Drinks can be used between meals to curb appetite without elevating blood sugar. An energy drink that promotes proper pH also aids in detoxification, but it's important the drink is free of sugar, artificial sweeteners and is low calorie.

A Daily Multi-Vitamin and Multi-Mineral with green tea, grape seed extract, cranberry extract, pomegranate extract, bioflavonoids, vitamins, minerals, herbs, antioxidants, digestive enzymes and probiotics is suggested. In addition to providing support for body systems during detoxing and for supplementing nutrition deficiencies from depleted soils, we like to see a high ORAC (Oxygen Free Radical Absorbent Capacity) score. An ORAC score of 10,000 is equivalent to eating 16 to 20 antioxidant packed fruits and vegetables.

Skincare

Use only hair, body and skin care products free of mineral oil, harmful chemicals, and additives.

Notes

Endnotes:

1 http://www.usc.edu/student-affairs/Health_Center/adolhealth/content/b3menses.
html#references

2 http://www.womentowomen.com/hormonalimbalance.aspx

3 http://66.241.252.6/images/femalehormon1.gif

4 Dr. John Lee, David Zava, Ph.D.: What Your Doctor May Not Tell You About Breast
Cancer. New York, Time Warner, 2002, p. 53.)

5 Giovanni Brambilla and Antonietta Martelli: Are some progestins genotoxic liver
carcinogens? Mutation Research/Reviews in Mutation Research, Volume 512, Issues
2-3, December 2002, Pages 155-163

6 A Bawde, WM Gregory, MA Chaudary et al,: Timing of surgery during menstrual
cycle and survival of premenopausal women with operable breast cancer, Lancet
1991 (337): 1261-1264. PE Mohr et al,: Serum progesterone levels at time of breast
surgery and long term survival in node positive patients, Brit J. Cancer 1996 (73):
1552-1555.

7 Georges J. M. Maestroni (1993) The immunoneuroendocrine role of melatonin
Journal of Pineal Research 14 (1) , 1–10 doi:10.1111/j.1600-079X.1993.tb00478.x

Further Reading:

Joseph Glenmullen, M.D. *The Antidepressant Solution: A Step-by-Step Guide to Safely Overcoming Antidepressant Withdrawal, Dependence, and "Addiction."* New York: Simon and Schuster, 2005.

Dr. John Lee and David Zava, Ph.D. *What Your Doctor May Not Tell You About Breast Cancer.* New York: Time Warner, 2002.

Dr. John Lee and Virginia Warner. *What Your Doctor May Not Tell You About Menopause.* New York: Warner Books, 2004.

David Perlmutter, M.D. and Carol Colman. *The Better Brain Book.* New York: Riverhead Books, 2004.

Barbara Seaman. *The Greatest Experiment Ever Performed on Women: Exploding the Estrogen Myth.* New York: Hyperion Books, 2003.

Suzanne Somers. *The Sexy Years.* New York: Crown Publishers, 2004.

Mark Hyman, M.D. and Mark Liponis, M.D. *Ultra-Prevention: The Six Week Plan That Will Make You Healthier For Life.* New York: Simon and Schuster, 2003.

Dr. Don Colbert. *Toxic Relief.* Lake Mary, Florida: Siloam Press, 2001.

Dr. Don Colbert. *The Seven Pillars of Health.* Lake Mary, Florida: Siloam Press, 2006.

Michael R. Eades, M.D. and Mary Dan Eades, M.D. *Protein Power: The High-Protein/ Low-Carbohydrate Way to Lose Weight, Feel Fit, and Boost Your Health – In Just Weeks!* New York: Bantam Books, 1999.

Toni Weschler. *Taking Charge of Your Fertility: The Definitive Guide to Natural Birth Control, Pregnancy Achievement, and Reproductive Health.* New York: Harper Collins, 2002

James Wilson. *Adrenal Fatigue – The 21st Century Stress Syndrome.* Petaluma, CA: Smart Publications, 2001.

Helpful Websites:

www.wholefoodmarkets.com
A wealth of information, do your research, make lists, get recipes, learn more or pre-shop before you enter the store

www.traderjoes.com
Informative, educational, get recipes, or pre-shop before going

www.foodforlife.com

www.foodshouldtastegood.com

www.ushealthfoodstores.com (find a store in your local area/state)

www.arbonne.com
Vegan and organic products for the whole body

www.foxhollowfarms.com
Grass-fed Beef - Louisville, KY area

www.zrtlabs.com
Saliva and blood spot testing